HEALTH MANPOWER:
PLANNING, PRODUCTION AND MANAGEMENT

This book reports on a study of the health manpower process within the British National Health Service. It explores manpower planning, production and management aims, methodologies and practices, and assesses their compatibility with the World Health Organization's 'Health for All by the Year 2000' strategy. It provides extensive reviews of the professional and official literature and details an investigative survey of manpower practices within District Health Authorities. Throughout, the book focuses upon medical, nursing and allied health practitioners. The orientation is towards the politics of health manpower, examining issues from the formulation of policy and technical details of the health manpower process, through to implementation and evaluation. In addition, three case studies of service innovations and their manpower implications are explored, namely: the development of community care for the mentally handicapped; teamwork in a health centre; and an expanded role for the nurse, in particular the potential of a nurse practitioner. The study concludes by developing an evaluative checklist of issues encompassing the health manpower process. The book will be of interest to health professionals, administrators, planners and managers, and to those concerned with the study of health services.

HEALTH MANPOWER:

PLANNING, PRODUCTION AND MANAGEMENT

ANDREW F. LONG and GEOFFREY MERCER

In collaboration with:
FIONA BROOKS
STEPHEN HARRISON
TOM RATHWELL
KEITH BARNARD

CROOM HELM
London • New York • Sydney

© 1987 Andrew F. Long and Geoffrey Mercer
Croom Helm Ltd, Provident House, Burrell Row,
Beckenham, Kent, BR3 1AT
Croom Helm Australia, 44-50 Waterloo Road,
North Ryde, 2113, New South Wales

British Library Cataloguing in Publication Data

Long, A.F.
  Health manpower: planning, production
  and management.
  1. Medical personnel — Great Britain —
  Supply and demand 2. Manpower — Planning
  — Great Britain
  I. Title II. Mercer, G.
  331.11'913621'0941   RA410.9.G7
  ISBN 0-7099-4172-2

Published in the USA by
Croom Helm
in association with Methuen, Inc.
29 West 35th Street
New York, NY 10001

Library of Congress Cataloging-in-Publication Data

ISBN 0-7099-4172-2

Printed and bound in Great Britain by
Biddles Ltd, Guildford and King's Lynn

CONTENTS

Abbreviations
Editorial Note
List of Contributors
Preface by J.-P. Menu, M.D.
Acknowledgements

ABBREVIATIONS

A and C	Administrative and Clerical Staff
ADSCP	Association of District and Superintendent Chartered Physiotherapists
ACMMP	Advisory Committee on Medical Manpower Planning
AHA	Area Health Authority
AHP	Allied Health Professional
ARP	Annual Review Process
BAOT	British Association of Occupational Therapists
BDA	British Dental Association
BGS	British Geriatrics Society
BMA	British Medical Association
CMC	Central Manpower Committee
CNO	Chief Nursing Officer
CPME	Council for Postgraduate Medical Education
CPSM	Council for Professions Supplementary to Medicine
CSP	Chartered Society of Physiotherapy
DDRB	Review Body on Doctors' and Dentists' Remuneration
DEB	Dental Estimates Board
DHA	District Health Authority
DHSS	Department of Health and Social Security
DMO	District Medical Officer
DMS	Director of Midwifery Services
DMT	District Management Team
DNS	Director of Nursing Services
DPO	District Personnel Officer
ENB	English National Board for Nursing, Midwifery and Health Visiting

Abbreviations

FPC	Family Practitioner Committee
FPS	Family Practitioner Service(s)
GDP	General Dental Practitioner
GMC	General Medical Council
GP	General Practitioner
HFA 2000	Health for All by the Year 2000
HMD	Health Manpower Development
HMP	Health Manpower Planning
JCHT/SAC	Joint Committee on Higher Training/ Specialty Advisory Committee
JCPTGP	Joint Committee on Postgraduate Training for General Practice
LEA	Local Education Authority
MEC	Medical Executive Committee
MIND	National Association for Mental Health
MLSO	Medical Laboratory Scientific Officer
MPAG	Manpower Planning Advisory Group
MPC	Medical Practices Committee
NHS	National Health Service
NP	Nurse Practitioner
OT	Occupational Therapist
PHC	Primary Health Care
PIs	Performance Indicators
PSM	Profession(s) Supplementary to Medicine
P and T	Professional and Technical Staff
RCCS	Revenue Consequences of Capital Schemes
RCGP	Royal College of General Practitioners
RHA	Regional Health Authority
RMC	Regional Medical Committee
RNTC	Regional Nurse Training Committee
RSCN	Registered Sick Childrens' Nurse
SASP	Summary Analysis of Strategic Plans
SEN	State Enrolled Nurse
SHHD	Scottish Home and Health Department
SRN	State Registered Nurse
STAMP	Standard Manpower Planning and Personnel Information System
UGC	University Grants Committee

Abbreviations

UKCC	United Kingdom Central Council for Nursing, Midwifery and Health Visiting
UMT	Unit Management Team
WHO	World Health Organization

EDITORIAL NOTE

This text is based on a research report on health manpower practices within the British health services. The one year study was funded by the European Office of the World Health Organization. A short synopsis of the original report has already been published as: <u>Investigating Practices in Health Manpower Planning: Report on a Country Case Study</u> (World Health Organization, Regional Office for Europe, ICP/HMD 101/501, Copenhagen, 1986).

The study was carried out under the general direction of A.F. Long who acted as the Principal Investigator. Full-time research assistance was provided by F. Brooks. Contributions to the project were also made in varying degrees by T. Rathwell, S. Harrison, K. Barnard and G. Mercer. The original report compiled by this group was completed and submitted to WHO in July 1985.

In order to present the material in book form, that report hs been significantly altered and extended. This work has been undertaken by A.F. Long and G. Mercer. A major difference entailed the imposition of a 'health manpower process' framework so as to provide a unifying and facilitating structure. It also required re-writing, together with the addition of material relevant to health manpower practices that has become available in the subsequent year. As some of the changes were substantial it has become impossible to neatly match author(s) with specific chapters. Allowing for the editing and re-writing introduced throughout the text by A.F. Long and G. Mercer, the following took the initial responsibility for writing up the material which appears in the current arrangement of chapters: Chapter 1, K. Barnard; Chapter 2, A.F. Long; Chapter 3, T. Rathwell and A.F. Long; Chapter 4, G. Mercer; Chapter 5, F. Brooks; Chapter 6, S. Harrison; Chapter 7, F. Brooks, A.F. Long and G. Mercer; Chapter 8, T. Rathwell; Chapters 9 to 11, F. Brooks; and Chapter 12, A. F. Long and

Editorial Note

G. Mercer.
Needless to say, we take the final responsibility for the material as presented here.

Andrew F. Long   University of Leeds
Geoffrey Mercer   December 1986

LIST OF CONTRIBUTORS

ANDREW F. LONG
Senior Research Fellow
School of Education
University of Leeds

GEOFFREY MERCER
Lecturer in Sociology
Department of Sociology
University of Leeds

FIONA BROOKS
(formerly) Research Assistant
Nuffield Centre
Department of Social Policy
and Health Services Studies
University of Leeds

STEPHEN HARRISON
Lecturer in Health Services Organisation
Nuffield Centre
Department of Social Policy
and Health Services Studies
University of Leeds

TOM RATHWELL
Lecturer in Health Planning
Nuffield Centre
Department of Social Policy
and Health Services Studies
University of Leeds

KEITH BARNARD
Senior Lecturer in Health Planning
Nuffield Centre
Department of Social Policy
and Health Services Studies
University of Leeds

PREFACE

Health manpower is an essential component of health services which can account for up to 80% of health expenditures in countries of Europe. It is therefore easy to understand why - in these times of financial dilemmas - health managers and policy-makers want to have a better understanding of how the planning, administration and deployment of health professionals can lead to more efficient delivery of health care.

At the same time, the development and spread of the European Health for All (HFA) policy offers new viewpoints from which to assess the manpower situation in a given country. This policy was worked out by the countries of the European Region of the World Health Organization (WHO) and endorsed by them in 1984. Based on the worldwide HFA goal, the policy calls for major shifts in the organisation and context of health care so that health promotion, disease prevention, and diagnostic, therapeutic and rehabilitative care can be used in the most effective and equitable way possible to meet the health needs of communities.

If HFA is to become a reality, changes in the planning, education, training and utilisation of health manpower are urgently needed to ensure appropriate delivery of health care. These changes call for concerted action among the various authorities responsible for the development of health services and health manpower. WHO sees as one of its main roles the promotion of such collaboration at national and subnational levels as well as suggesting alternative approaches for adapting the health manpower process to the HFA strategy.

In 1984, the European Office of WHO approached the Nuffield Centre at the University of Leeds, as a WHO collaborating centre, in order to develop and test a methodological approach for analysing the

health manpower development process in a given
area. Through a one year pilot study, the Nuffield
Centre established a methodology and applied it to
an examination of health manpower practices in
Britain. The study had three objectives: to
identify and describe existing health manpower
practices, to examine their compatibility with the
European HFA strategy and to explore some specific
practices supporting HFA.

The results are very informative. It was
comparatively easy to research hospital based
services on which much information is available.
Exploring current and potential developments in
primary health care was more complex, but the
research team was able to analyse several success
stories whose common denominator was to view the
primary health care approach as a way to promote as
well as to preserve health.

This publication is an extension of the
original study report submitted to WHO. The views
expressed are those of the authors and do not
necessarily represent the stated policy of the
World Health Organisation. Broad dissemination of
the results of the study is, nevertheless, of
considerable importance to WHO, as this is one of
the very rare occasions where actual practices in
health manpower planning and management are
identified in some amount of detail and in relation
to the HFA strategy.

As for the future, the methodology developed
through the study will be further tested and
applied for exploring manpower issues in other
Member States. Simultaneously, the experience
gained will be used to identify health manpower
implications of the Regional health strategy and to
outline a number of scenarios for health manpower.
It is hoped that such 'guiding principles' will be
expanded progressively and strengthen the policy-
making processes of the Member States.

J.-P. Menu, MD
Regional Officer for Health Manpower Development
WHO Regional Office for Europe

ACKNOWLEDGEMENTS

Grateful acknowledgement is made to the European Office of the World Health Organization for funding the study, and especially Dr. A. Wojtczak, and Dr. J.-P. Menu.

Carrying out a postal questionnaire survey and an interview based study involves the support and assistance of many persons; to all the respondents in the NHS, who willingly gave up their time to assist us, we are grateful. Particular mention must be made of the following: Miss B.M. Folkard and Mr D. Donald; Sister B. Stilwell; Mr S. Robbins; Dr J. Sinson; and all the staff at the health centre, especially Dr M. Walsh.

Finally, many thanks are extended to Carole Munro. She, with support from Sarah Barklam, has pursued the document through its many redrafts in the final report to this book.

Andrew F. Long
Geoffrey Mercer

University of Leeds
December, 1986

Chapter 1

HEALTH MANPOWER: THE WHO CONTEXT

In October 1984, the World Health Organization (WHO) held an inter-regional consultation on Health Manpower Development (HMD) in Jakarta, Indonesia (WHO, 1986). The objectives of the meeting were:

. to identify and clarify the issues which needed to be addressed;
. to generate useable models for decision makers and others involved;
. to develop relevant national or local manpower policies; and
. to translate these into practical plans.

The issue of implementation was the central focus. This implied that manpower planning had already reached a desirable level of sophistication. The problems lay elsewhere in the production of manpower with the appropriate competences by the various education and training institutions and programmes, and in their subsequent deployment and utilisation by the health services, that is, manpower management. Whatever the validity of such a judgement on the quality of manpower planning methodology, the analyses presented by participants suggested that HMD was still awaiting strategies which would rescue it from existing professional provider interests and integrate it into the framework of national and local health policy. It remains uncomfortably true that in many health systems decisions on manpower are one way or another kept in the hands of provider interests and are constructed on their view of broader health policy which is then rationalised in such a way as to be publicly presentable while guarding self-interest as effectively as possible.

The Jakarta group was presented with a selection of HMD pathologies. These were synthesised into three broad areas labelled:

1

1 **administration and management:**
   this led to proposals for ensuring improved
   internal procedures within a given health
   service agency for creating and filling
   posts, for more purposeful dealings with
   superior and subordinate bodies wherever it
   was necessary to involve them.

2 **education and training:**
   this generated guidance on bringing the
   suppliers of trained manpower into a more
   sustained dialogue with the users of their
   output, the health service institutions to
   seek some mutually acceptable assessment of
   the 'need' for manpower, the prerequisites
   of personal qualities and educational
   attainment to be observed in selecting
   trainees, and the competences, values and
   behaviour to be imparted to them and be
   demonstrable on completion of training. The
   example was cited of rejection by
   'autonomous' universities, and particularly
   their medical schools of requests from
   government health departments to train new
   kinds of health workers, citing academic
   freedom as the justification.

3 **political and organisational:**
   this embraced the need for political and
   leadership skills at the head of the HMD
   function. It was necessary to secure and
   maintain the commitment of political
   decision makers, to build up an effective
   coherent organisation, to negotiate
   successfully with other bodies in the same
   and in other sectors and to maintain the
   support of all those involved in HMD, and
   not least to demonstrate both a sustained
   sense of purpose and a readiness to act
   pragmatically in the light of results and
   changed circumstances without losing that
   sense of purpose.

   Notwithstanding the very real efforts to come
to terms with problems and to make positive
proposals, the participants found themselves
fighting off two pervasive sentiments: cynicism
because nothing would be changed; or frustration
because it seemed that nothing could be changed.
For example, plans often had no reference to broader
health policy objectives, and policies were made
which had no realistic chance of being implemented.

WHO's engagement in the issue was perhaps of itself testimony that it was a difficult, almost intractable, problem that needed supranational effort to find a solution. The underlying issue - that of reorienting health systems - had been on WHO's agenda for a decade or longer. This can be unpacked to make explicit some very basic questions:

- . what should be the nature of health policy?
- . what are the consequences of the content of policy for the established health sector, especially medicine?
- . what are the implications in terms of the types and numbers of manpower and how are they to be produced? and
- . what should be the role of WHO in such matters?

As for the role of WHO as an international organisation, it exists to assist member states, to respond to their wishes and requests, and to provide technical support in such matters as epidemiology and disease control. Health policy, while it may have an international dimension (as in the flow of epidemiological intelligence), is an internal matter for member states. Likewise, so is the structure and scope of the health sector and the degree of control they choose to exercise over health sector manpower; the types of manpower they sanction; the mode of training and licensure; the measure of self-government they cede to organised bodies of health workers (archetypally physicians); whether for planning and budgetary purposes they might translate health policy into actual activities and the tasks to be carried out and by whom. The potential enormity of these issues is obvious, particularly when coupled with decision makers' reluctance to proceed until the costs of the consequences of inaction exceed the costs of action. Indeed, the enormity might well be thought of as sufficient grounds for not upsetting the existing modus vivendi with the various interests including established provider groups and departments of state other than health (for example, education), who may well be stakeholders in this particular arena. In fact, in relatively few member states does it appear to be the case that there is one government department able to formulate health policy in its widest sense, identify the manpower implications of that policy, and then act accordingly to plan numbers of each manpower category (defined by tasks to be done), to produce through education and training, and then to deploy and manage them. In most countries machinery exists which allows dialogue with providers of trained manpower. But that does not make it easier to modify the tasks of an existing manpower category or to introduce a new type of worker who will subsequently be a cheaper substitute to a well-established provider. On the other hand, it would appear that in some member states the possibility of such a dialogue does not exist. In such political cultures, its legitimacy is not acknowledged.

Whatever the propensities and possibilities of health departments to formulate health policies and follow through the manpower implications, there will be a pool of trained manpower, replenished by the output of various training programmes. What happens by way of services provided will depend on their rewards and motivations, the distribution of tasks between different types of worker, the technical and psychological relationships between types of worker, the therapeutic efficacy of their skills and techniques, the match of those abilities to the 'needs' of the population, and the location of these workers in relation to the density of population served. In this way there is always a health manpower plan and, by extension, a health policy although they may both be implicit and by default.

One possible consequence of a laissez-faire approach to health manpower and hence health policy is the accelerated fragmentation of the therapeutic task into more and more sub-occupations each seeking formal recognition, enhanced status and, wherever possible, a monopoly position.

> 'In a simpler day the health professions consisted only of apothecaries ... surgeons ... and nurses .... Today attempts to list health occupations practised in the United States easily run into the hundreds' (Weisfeld, 1984, p. 66).

The writer goes on to identify various consequences including the extension of 'anti-trust' laws to break those groups seeking to establish a monopoly position.

'... Many observers fear anti-trust legislation as a pernicious influence on the development of rational and predictable health policy. Their apprehension is exploited by ... professional monopolies ... who stand to lose a great deal of privilege under an enthusiastic anti-trust regime' (ibid).

So if laissez-faire and the anti-trust response in the USA is likely to prove a false trail to rational health policy, are the signs in the European Region more encouraging? The report of the WHO Regional Conference on Primary Health Care (WHO, 1985a) records a search for positive indications. Primary health care (PHC) was seen as embracing prevention and promotion, the adaptation of technology to help people stay in familiar surroundings whenever and for as long as possible; in sum the integration of all aspects of care. But the report notes that health systems are generally not sensitive to the needs of individuals, families and communities and that medical training is preparation for hospital careers in many instances, while PHC teaching is rudimentary and isolated. It goes on to identify in a deceptively simple way what is needed by way of information: the demographic variables, the health status of the population, the prevailing health problems, the environmental risk factors, the present usage of resources, information on legislation and policy changes and the development of qualitative indicators. As for manpower it argued for the following:

. the case for recognising a specialty of general medical practice or primary care physicians. While there is an actual and forecast glut of physicians, this masks a shortage of general medical practitioners;
. entrants to this specialty should do so more positively and not reluctantly;
. the principles of PHC should also be taught to students in law, engineering, economics and other non-medical sciences, recognising the multiple interests involved in PHC; and
. care should not just be left to the established health care professions. There is a case for new kinds of workers in home community care with courses for lay people in fields such as cardio-pulmonary

resuscitation, accident prevention and nursing.

Clearly the territory is rich in potential controversy both in problem definition and alternative strategies. A Health Minister may wonder whether some breaking of the rigid lines of demarcation is possible, and the trend to specialisation could be reversed. The Minister will perhaps sense the discontinuity between health policy which the government espouses and the rigidities of the professional labour supply. In addition, the Minister who has just come into office may well wonder what should be made of the philosophy of health policy articulated by WHO for and on behalf of member states and how it evolved the way it did.

Probably the first thing that will be pointed out, at least by detractors of the organisation, is that WHO is committed to a totally unrealistic view of health as a 'state of complete physical, mental and social well-being not merely the absence of disease or infirmity'. This could mean that health services are laying claim to everything (Strong, 1986). Article 1 of WHO's constitution states: 'the objective of WHO shall be the attainment by all peoples of the world of the highest possible level of health'. Striving after the possible is not unrealistic, although how to interpret the Article is a matter of dispute. In its early years the WHO secretariat interpreted its remit in a narrow technical sense and aroused no controversy. It was largely confined to the dissemination of technical, including epidemiological, information and the provision of technical assistance. By the 1970s this situation was changing fast. Newly independent developing countries dominated WHO membership. Across the international agencies there was an enhanced awareness of the circumstances of the populations of these new states, and the problems of meeting their basic needs including health.

The work on analysing and clarifying these needs and ways of responding continued through the 1970s and climaxed in two key events. First, in 1977, the annual global health parliament, the World Health Assembly of delegations of all member states, passed a resolution committing these states to seeking as a major social goal 'Health For All by the Year 2000' (HFA 2000). Notwithstanding the prophetic ring in the phrase, the intention was to generate political momentum for a positive health policy in all member states, a more active popular involvement through community participation, and more and better distributed human and other resources going to the health sector to be used to attack major community health problems. It was clear that this would involve joint action with other sectors - agriculture, education, transport, industry and so on - and so community participation and inter-sectoral action were identified as necessary conditions for HFA. The objective of HFA was not to attempt to put the lid back on Pandora's Box but more prosaically to enable all citizens 'to lead socially and economically productive lives'.

The second key event came in 1978 with the International Conference (WHO/UNICEF) at Alma Ata, USSR, which endorsed the concept of primary health care as the means of promoting better health in populations (WHO, 1978). This concept of PHC was distinguished from the more traditional notion of primary medical care. PHC includes local first contact services with primary physicians and other community based health workers. These services are identified as the first point in a national system of patient referral to increasingly complex and technically sophisticated services of diagnosis, treatment, care and rehabilitation, according to the individual's needs. But PHC also embraces all health-related activities, such as safe water and sanitation, adequate food supply and proper nutrition, and a healthy physical environment, together with public information and education on health problems. When properly organised and co-ordinated with medical care, all such elements of PHC contribute to the management of health promotion and disease prevention and control.

This comprehensive approach to health will involve a country's health sector in a range of initiatives, some new, and some strengthening or amending existing activities. It will also most importantly involve the health sector in seeking and obtaining the willing co-operation of the responsible agencies in other sectors whose activities can have a positive effect on the population's health: hence an emphasis on inter-sectoral action such as with agriculture, manufacturing industry, transport, housing, education and social welfare. Equally, there is an emphasis on community participation, not only in planning and managing services by whatever means are customary and appropriate, but in underlining people's personal responsibility for their own

health.
    Subsequent to the Alma Ata Conference, member states as assisted by the WHO Secretariat have been pursuing these fundamental policy objectives through the development of HFA strategies. At the European Regional Committee in 1980, a Regional Strategy was adopted. Following the PHC approach the Strategy has three main thrusts:

    . the promotion of healthier life styles;
    . the reduction of avoidable risks and hazards to health; and
    . the provision of accessible comprehensive health services through PHC.

These principles were further elaborated (WHO, 1985b), and 38 health related objectives or 'targets' were identified and the ways in which they could be achieved.
    The targets document develops from two basic assertions: despite the resources made available and the scale of technical advances related to health, firstly the level of health of populations is lower than it could be and secondly significant inequalities in health remain both within and between countries. The Regional targets are therefore expressed as proposed concrete action in attacking health problems, seeking improvements in health and taking the necessary enabling measures. They are intended to stimulate and assist member states in setting national targets which will reflect needs, priorities and values. An analysis of the 38 targets shows that they can be clustered in the following way:

    . those relating to the general principles of the Regional Strategy and creating the necessary conditions for improving the health of populations and reducing inequities;
    . those relating to essential support measures as in information and management arrangements, mechanisms for policy implementation and the allocation of resources;
    . those relating to the development of trained manpower, committed to the PHC approach, with the necessary competences both to deal with the main health problems of the population and as appropriate to ensure quality of care;

- a relevant health research strategy to match the main body of operational targets directed at identified health problems;
- operational targets, that is, statements of objectives and measures required in order to promote health, to reduce the incidence of disease, and to create a healthy environment; and
- the development and use of appropriate technology in diagnosis and treatment.

It is intended that member states will use and adapt these targets according to their particular circumstances. These will include the existing level of development of appropriate policies, services and other measures, the scale and nature of particular problems, the social and cultural context in which initiatives will be taken, the prevailing economic climate and the political and organisational arrangements.

In the course of its exposition the targets document notes a number of manpower issues including the importance of aligning manpower with the substantive health policy objectives. From the European Regional perspective it is evident that much remains to be done in all phases of HMD - in planning, production and management. There are major challenges with manpower outside the health sector if intersectoral action is to be at all feasible. But a start must be made within the health sector. The Jakarta meeting is a measure of how much needs to be done; it also raises questions of what it is possible to do.

Chapter 2

INVESTIGATING THE HEALTH MANPOWER PROCESS

The previous chapter has set out a number of issues
and challenges being faced in the European Region of
WHO concerning health manpower development, and
identified health targets adopted by all member
states in the Region. It is now apposite to enquire
as to what the exact state of the art is in terms of
current manpower practices, potentials and
innovations, and attempts being made, if any, to
mitigate and overcome constraining factors which
otherwise might inhibit the achievement of the
targets for HFA 2000. This chapter delineates a
methodology to explore the various dimensions of
HMD. In particular, three areas are examined:

- how to investigate current practices
  and associated constraining factors;
- how to investigate practices which could be
  identified as being compatible and
  supportive to HFA 2000; and
- how to investigate the manpower implications
  of HFA and the associated target document
  (WHO, 1985b), that is future manpower
  requirements.

In so doing the objectives and approach adopted
within the British study of health manpower
practices will be outlined. However, as a
preliminary it is important to clarify the content
and thrust of health manpower development.

THE HEALTH MANPOWER PROCESS

Mejia (1978) speaks of 'the health manpower process'
with respect to health manpower development. This
has three dimensions: planning, production and
management. Looking first of all at the health
manpower planning dimension (HMP), its aim is

'... to design manpower mixes and utilisation patterns in order to move the health manpower system from a given situation to a predetermined improved situation' (p.35).

This dimension is however not only concerned with formulating plans, but also with their implementation. The general objective is 'to specify the number of teams and the composition, needed to improve the level of health up to a proposed level' (see Table 2.1).

A number of questions can then be raised. Firstly, what is meant by a 'health team'? Indeed, are 'health manpower teams' the centre of attention in actual manpower planning, or is it rather the number of physicians, nurses, and other professions allied to medicine which are specified? The link of such teams and/or manpower groups to meeting specific service objectives is also an important area to clarify. Secondly, the objective of HMP clearly points to a link between manpower input and health outcome. This raises the issue of the state of knowledge over the population's health and available health manpower in general, for specific groups, and as teams providing a service, and over the effectiveness of the service provided. Thirdly, it also suggests the importance of outlining desirable characteristics for the members of the teams (the health manpower workforce) in terms, say, of qualifications, experience, age, gender, and so on. Such questions as these need resolution prior to the production of the manpower and also for its effective management and use.

The production dimension is concerned with '... all aspects related to the basic and post-basic education and training of the health labour force' (p.37). But while production is one of the central aspects of the health manpower process it is not under the control of the health system. Indeed, depending on the national context and also the professional groups themselves, the health system will have more or less influence.

'The fragmentation of control and this diversity of interests (health educational institutions, professional associations and health system) lead educational institutions to tend to act with little regard to the existence of health and manpower plans....' (p.38).

Table 2.1: The Health Manpower Process

	Health Manpower Planning	Health Manpower Production	Health Manpower Management
Central Objective	to specify the number of teams and the composition needed to improve the level of health up to a proposed level	to produce x people of y types	to determine manpower distribution and productivity standards, patterns of utilisation and non-labour inputs
Specific Objectives	*to formulate health manpower plans and establish mechanisms for their implementation *to influence health manpower production *to ensure continuing staff development and the most effective possible distribution and use of existing manpower resources *to establish a monitoring system for the ongoing evaluation of manpower plans	*to produce the required numbers and types of staff *to ensure that the training and education curricula match the requirements of the health system	*to recruit persons with desirable characteristics (monitor manpower requirements) *to use manpower effectively (utilisation policies) *to motivate manpower (incentives, career development, performance evaluation) *to reduce staff turnover
Target	x health teams of y composition in operation by time t	x trained personnel of y type by time t	x units of service of specified quality delivered to a defined population
Comment	an optimising process	need for co-ordination and integration with health manpower planing and managment	organic relationship to the health manpower process as a whole: manpower requirements are based on utilisation patterns which determine educational objectives ...

Source: adapted from Mejia, 1978, Table 1 'The Scope of the Health Manpower Process', p.36.

The critical task of health planners to ensure co-ordination and integration can be seen, thus reiterating the objective of the production dimension, 'to produce x people of y type'.

The production component embraces manpower supply in general: that is, education of new recruits, retraining and continuing education for current and potential members of the workforce, policies for retention (for those with 'desirable characteristics') and policies on general recruitment. It should be noted that whether or not a team approach to HMP has been adopted, attention will centre in the production dimension on the generation of individual health workers by professional groups and rarely of teams of health workers, at least given current education and training practices.

The final dimension of the health manpower process is that of management, which

'... covers all matters related to employment, use, and motivation of all categories of health workers, and largely determines the productivity, and therefore the coverage, of the health services system and its capacity to retain staff' (p.39).

Optimising the use of the available health manpower is the aim: that is, a concern with equity, effectiveness and efficiency. Here again, the complicating issue of professionalism emerges. Questions of the current, appropriate and potential role of health workers, and the possibility of substitution and role enlargement in situations of labour shortage need to be raised, in addition to searching for ways to maximise health output for a given manpower (and other) input. The target of the management dimension of the health manpower process should be noted: 'x units of service of specified quality delivered to a defined population'. This reference to the quality of care brings discussion full circle back to the objective of HMP.

Each of these dimensions - planning, production and management - is interdependent. Projections of manpower requirements tend to be based on current utilisation patterns themselves influencing educational institutions and resulting training and education. The keynote to any match of the needs of the health system, its development, and the education of the health professionals lies therefore in co-ordination across the dimensions of the health manpower process. Their integration, together with health services planning, both inter and intrasectorally, has to be a major emphasis. There is however an almost inevitable degree of tension between the dimensions. The education sector seeks to establish independence, to impose higher standards and to pursue greater specialisation (the pursuit of the best qualified with the most specific knowledge). This receives added support from the relevant professional associations (an increase in professional status). The management sector, especially in a climate of restriction over resources, is left to pursue control policies (over cost, numbers and so on) which are directed especially towards the more vulnerable manpower groups to the extent of potentially ignoring the actual delivery of care and its quality. The planning dimension is left almost in a void, either painting ideals for service delivery and manpower (teams) or generating plans with little commitment or hope of implementation. Who then in the organisation has the task of ensuring integration and co-ordination across the three dimensions of the health manpower process?

The essential political nature of the health manpower process must therefore be noted. As Mejia observes,

'... a wide variety of forces, constraints, and confrontations between organisations that have historically pursued their own objectives are involved' (p.53).

The three dimensions, each overlapping a further aspect comprising the 'development of the health services', are pulling away from one another, whereas the need is for them to draw together and work towards a common goal, the development of the health services for HFA 2000 (cf Fulop, 1976).

Against this background, how then can health manpower practices be investigated? As a sine qua non, it becomes essential to review a country's health manpower process - that is, planning, production, and management - and integrative and co-ordinating mechanisms, and issues of implementation and evaluation. In addition, such a review must both describe the current situation and consider how it might be changed to lead to an improved position. Thus the aim is to challenge the current state of affairs in a constructive vein, to lead to appropriate health services development, in the interests of the consumers of health services and not solely the professionals.

CURRENT PRACTICES

The starting point for any investigation of the health manpower process, integration mechanisms and constraints, is a review of current practices. In this regard a number of approaches suggest themselves, namely:

- reviewing the relevant professional and academic literature;
- interviewing actors within the manpower process;
- interviewing those within relevant professional associations; and
- assessing appropriate documents, plans and implementation papers, curricula and the like.

Each of the above strategies would need to be pursued in relation to the major sectors of the health services: for example, the primary health care context and hospital services. In addition, it is necessary to embrace, as appropriate, both the publicly and privately funded health services, drawing out the tensions between them in relation to health manpower, its training and education, recruitment, pay levels and so on.

Looking firstly at the literature review, a number of sources need to be examined in order to gain a complete and thorough overview of the relevant methodologies used: for example, to estimate manpower requirements; the attention given to the production and training of manpower; and concerns with issues such as the career structure, the tendency to greater specialisation, maldistribution of manpower and improper utilisation patterns. There are the writings of the professionals themselves in journals as well as more extensive accounts in texts and academic books. In addition, there are the publications of the relevant ministries (health, employment and education) and guidance over manpower given to Health Authorities and institutions involved in the education of health personnel, drawn up by ministries, other tiers in the health service organisation, and professional groups themselves. Throughout, it is critical not only to assess the methodologies used and key issues, but also to get behind the 'official' rhetoric to the ways things really are planned, produced and managed, and to see who is involved in the planning and policy making process. So, for example, who are the actors who actually determine the numbers to enter medical schools, on what criteria are these decided, whose interests are advanced, and so on?

This leads onto the second and third approaches of interviewing relevant personnel in the area. Two main groups of persons present themselves: actors involved in the planning, production or management processes at the many tiers in the health service (national, Regional, District, Unit); and officers within the relevant professional groups who are, or could be, significant actors in determining plans, working practices, utilisation patterns and the like. As wide a range of persons should be talked to in the several ministries involved, the professions and the local Health Authorities. Again, the concern is to get behind the apparent decision making process to discern the latent workings and actors involved within the field.

Finally, the actual plans and their implementation, and other official documents of the local Health Authority in particular and of other levels in the health setting must be reviewed. Both strategic (long term) and operational (the immediate implementation) plans need to be examined, and preferably a series of such documents relating both to the past as well as the future. Stated planning intentions can then be compared with proposed actions and eventual implementation; these also would form a useful background for the later questioning of the relevant actors.

Through the pursuit of the above approaches, a fairly complete picture of current practices in the area of health manpower can be identified, as well as constraints and limitations to integration or in implementing plans. Of course, it may be the case because of time, money or manpower that not all of them can be pursued; indeed, only a sample of the possible actors can be interviewed either face to face or through the use of a postal questionnaire. In this instance concern must be to ensure that the persons interviewed are representative. It must be stressed that the most difficult problem to overcome is to obtain insight into the latent decision making and planning process, and not to remain at the level of the manifest official position.

SUPPORTIVE PRACTICES

The fundamental question to be addressed prior to any investigation at this level is that of, 'what is a supportive practice?' In the context of this text the guiding orientation is that of the HFA 2000 and the associated targets document (WHO, 1985b). Accordingly, given its emphasis on a reorientation of services to primary health care, manpower practices which might be seen as supportive or compatible with such a strategy are then the focus of study. The adoption of a multi-disciplinary team approach to the provision of PHC, a concern with health promotion at the PHC level, and the like, need to be examined with particular emphasis on their manpower implications: for example, how were such innovations set up, what was their rationale, how and what decisions were made on skills required, and so on? In addition, criteria used to review and judge current practices could be employed to identify initiatives and innovations which overcome some of the constraints and limitations surrounding them or which possess desirable features.

The particular target associated with HMD in the HFA document reads as follows:

'Before 1990, in all Member States, the planning, training and use of health personnel should be in accordance with health for all policies, with emphasis on the primary health care approach.

This can be achieved if all countries analyse their need for the different categories of health manpower required to implement their policies of health for all, adopt suitable health manpower policies, and decide on the numbers and educational qualifications required for each category of personnel' (Target 36, WHO, 1985b).

As the accompanying text identifies, this points towards several salient aspects to review and evaluate current manpower practices, namely:

. within the health system, does planning reflect needs: that is, is there a correspondence between academic training goals and service requirements, consumer expectations and the general socio-economic situation? (ibid, p.141)

- is there a co-ordinated training and education programme for health personnel, leading to the right numbers of individuals with the right qualifications to meet the needs specified? (p. 142)
- are the training and education programmes relevant to PHC? For, training programmes should aim '... to satisfy the health needs and demands of individuals and communities and not primarily conform to professional interests.... Teaching should be ... community oriented and should pay close attention to local health promotive, preventive, curative and rehabilitative activities' (p.143).
- are there programmes of continuing education to develop practising health professionals, and to bring their work more closely in line with the health needs of the population? This leads onto an emphasis on PHC and teamwork (p.144).

From reviewing Target 36 for HFA and literature on the theory and practice of health manpower a characterisation of ideal practice can be drawn up. The planning, production and management dimensions of the health manpower process, strategies for integration and constraints must form the focus of any list of criteria. An attempt can be made to create such a list both in terms of what practitioners at the various monitoring levels in the health service perceive, and in terms of what might be deemed desirable characteristics within the relevant literature. Once a set have been delineated their usefulness in reviewing current practices and in identifying supportive practices is apparent. In addition, they can be used to elucidate the ways potential manpower initiatives and innovations may be constrained.

INVESTIGATING FUTURE MANPOWER REQUIREMENTS

A change in orientation is involved in exploring future manpower requirements, moving from a position of reviewing current practices and innovations and constraining factors, and from establishing and employing criteria to evaluate such practices. Indeed, its reference point is wider, to the future state of health care. Discerning required manpower skills and ways in which they should be deployed in accordance with any emerging shift in health care is no easy task: the mix of skills presently appertaining is quite likely to be different from that required in the future. Taking HFA as the guide to the shape of future health care, this strategy implies a reorientation of the current concept, in particular towards PHC.

A first step is to question perceived requirements and to attempt to evaluate their appropriateness given current health manpower plans. This inevitably involves a critical review of the mechanisms for integration. For example, it may be possible to achieve a desired future state of health provision by changing utilisation patterns (the management dimension), having extensive discussions with relevant professions and the associations in order 'to redirect current practices. Or, trying to exercise or expand influence over the educational sector may be apposite (the production dimension). The very fact that change may foster resistance is not a reason for maintaining the status quo. The thorough investigation of current practices of health manpower planning, production and management, integrative aspects and constraints, as well as an exploration of the political networks, forms an essential building block for any challenging of current manpower practices and the exploration of future requirements.

With HFA as a background, more far reaching developments are suggested. The Regional Strategy points out that not only will roles and responsibilities alter, but also new types and combinations of skilled and semi-skilled manpower may be necessary. The difficulty is determining what configurations of manpower are required. There is a need for a system or procedure which enables a range of possible futures to be considered and events tailored or planned in a relevant fashion. One such method is that of scenario writing. A wide range of approaches and styles are available in this mode.

Two broad types can be distinguished: end or beginning state driven, and mainly environmentally or mainly actor driven. The first type signifies whether the scenario writer started with the present and worked forward to the future, or specified the future a priori and worked through to determine how it can or will be achieved (Hirschorn, 1980). The second type, itself more of a continuum than a dichotomy, is concerned with the emphasis given by the scenario writer to factors outside of the control of actors in the situation compared to those within their sphere of influence. Those for whom the environment is of prime importance may employ models in which a number of environmental factors are assumed to account for most of the important variations in the future. The user of the scenario can then decide how to react so as to minimise the effect of the environment upon the organisation. In contrast, those variables that can be influenced or manipulated by the actors can be addressed: the more factors open to manipulation the more proactive the user can be.

The type of approach to choose depends on one's objectives. Given the backcloth of HFA 2000, a beginning driven scenario would be rejected as it is based on current practices which may not be of themselves consonant with HFA. In contrast, the questioning of current practices could indeed adopt such an approach. Accordingly, the most appropriate method is one that takes account of the major environmental constraints in the health context - for example, finance, the extent of health care provided, and the type of education and training currently undertaken - and explores both how to take these trends into account and how to modify them in order to bring about the desired future of HFA: that is, the second type of approach. This would allow one to construct a range of questions such as:

'what types of workers are suggested? What skills and expertise are needed? Do such workers exist now? Do new types of workers need to be developed? Can existing types be modified? And what are the basic and continuing educational implications of these questions?' (Rathwell, Long and Harrison, 1985, p.14).

The use of the method of scenario writing would help to address the health and non-health manpower issues, factors surrounding the production of manpower (basic and continuing education and training), and potential barriers and obstacles in achieving HFA 2000 through PHC. Both challenging current practices, and postulating a desirable future, provide a valuable approach to build upon the investigation of current manpower practices, and possible criteria of evaluation in order to develop a desired health service.

THE BRITISH STUDY: AIMS AND METHODOLOGY

The above discussion has attempted to outline how

health manpower can be investigated in general, within the context of the theoretical frame of reference of the health manpower process, and the need for integration of its elements. Attention now turns to the translation of this conceptual approach into an empirical study of health manpower practices.

At the behest of the WHO Regional Office for Europe, to assist in the exploration and development of health manpower issues, a study was undertaken at the University of Leeds, which reviewed current practices in the health manpower field within the British National Health Service (NHS). It was established as a pilot study in terms of methodology and findings, for later extension to other countries. The one year study (April 1984 to 1985) had three aims:

. to identify and describe health manpower practices;
. to examine such practices against the aims of HFA 2000 with a view to their compatibility and supportiveness; and
. to investigate current health manpower practices perceived as being supportive to HFA.

The study's objectives were broad and inevitably had to be limited in scope given the timespan of the project. The overall rationale was to use the British pilot study as a reference point, given the complexity within the British system of the planning, production and management dimensions and their interaction, and in particular constraints to integration. Once a clarification of current manpower practices was obtained, the next step would be a concentration on the manpower requirements for HFA and on ways to achieve them within such a developed and politically bounded health and education system as Britain. The study reported on here is thus only a part of a longer term research activity.

To achieve the first objective and thus to draw up an inventory of approaches and methodologies employed in health manpower planning, it was essential to review both hospital based services (employing 91% of all National Health Service manpower) and primary health care services. A three pronged strategy as depicted in Figure 2.1 was applied, in order to glean details on the breadth of

Figure 2.1: An Overview of Methodology

A: Objective I - to identify and describe practices in HMD, and in particular HMP.

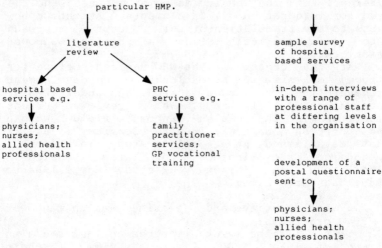

literature review

hospital based services e.g.

physicians;
nurses;
allied health
professionals

PHC services e.g.

family
practitioner
services;
GP vocational
training

sample survey
of hospital
based services

in-depth interviews
with a range of
professional staff
at differing levels
in the organisation

development of a
postal questionnaire
sent to

physicians;
nurses;
allied health
professionals

B: Objective II - to examine such strategies against the aims of HFA 2000

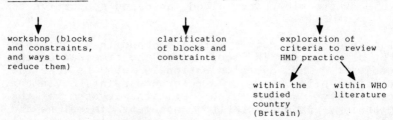

workshop (blocks
and constraints,
and ways to
reduce them)

clarification
of blocks and
constraints

exploration of
criteria to review
HMD practice

within the
studied
country
(Britain)

within WHO
literature

C: Objective III - to investigate current health manpower practices perceived as supportive to HFA 2000

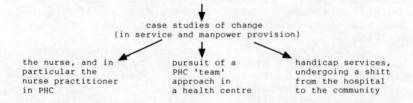

case studies of change
(in service and manpower provision)

the nurse, and in
particular the
nurse practitioner
in PHC

pursuit of a
PHC 'team'
approach in
a health centre

handicap services,
undergoing a shift
from the hospital
to the community

22

approaches.

Firstly, a review of recent professional literature for three of the major health providing groups - physicians, nurses and allied health professional workers - was undertaken. Its aim was to identify attention given in the literature to manpower planning and related issues, and specifically to issues relating to the role of the profession, methodologies for estimating manpower requirements and generating supply. In addition, to cast light on primary health care services, a review of past trends and current initiatives in relation to general medical practice was carried out. Issues explored included current and proposed service planning arrangements (financing the service, the Family Practitioner Committee (FPC), and its new planning role) and manpower issues (the role of the general practitioner and the primary health care team). A comprehensive historical literature review was not attempted: rather, concern lay with drawing out the relevant discussions within the professions to contrast with the survey findings on actual practice. The literature review thus set out to provide insight into the general context of health manpower planning, key issues and attitudes prior to an examination of actual Health Authority manpower planning practices.

Secondly, as a major part of the study, a sample survey investigation was carried out within hospital based services into current manpower practices and in particular the manpower planning and management dimensions of the health manpower process. As a starting point, a series of semi-structured interviews were undertaken with key actors in the management and planning field at a range of levels in the NHS (Region, District, and Unit) in a small number of Health Authorities. Building on this pilot interview survey, a postal questionnaire was drawn up and circulated to one in three District Health Authorities in England and Wales. Scotland and Northern Ireland were excluded from the study due to pressures of time and limitations of resources. A District focus was adopted because of their key role in the planning process, in both operational and strategic terms, considering long-term manpower demand and supply and its achievement, with the Region performing a co-ordinating and monitoring role. Details on the questionnaire and sampling are described below in Chapter Seven, which discusses the findings from this survey.

Taken together, the multiple methods employed to explore the first study objective were designed to cast differing but complementary light on current practices of health manpower planning in the British NHS. The literature review highlighted areas of concern within the professions, as well as methodologies for estimating manpower requirements. The survey data, while focussed only on hospital based manpower, exemplified the breadth of practice in planning and managing health manpower. The later exploration of case studies in PHC in pursuit of the third study objective provided a necessary extension to embrace health manpower practices across the primary and hospital sectors of the NHS.

The investigation of the second and third objectives was by no means straightforward. To assist in their exploration, a workshop on HFA and HMD was held, with representatives from the NHS and other European countries. Discussion concentrated upon verifying the findings arising from study of the first objective, and then upon the issue of blocks, difficulties and constraints to HMP, and potential ways to overcome them, within the context of reorienting health services towards PHC as a major thrust of the HFA 2000 strategy.

To further explore the second objective of the study - 'to examine such practices against the aims of HFA 2000 with a view to compatibility and supportiveness' - sets of criteria were constructed to review current manpower practices and to identify those of potential. In particular, strengths and weaknesses in emphasis in current health manpower practices were postulated. Secondly, blocks and challenges presented within the NHS and its associated professions to changes in role, numbers, and the like were elicited with a view to identifying their nature and form, and thus clarifying ways to surmount them.

Finally, to achieve the third objective - 'to investigate current practices perceived as supportive to HFA' - a series of case studies were carried out. These covered the following areas: planning for mental handicap services undergoing a shift from hospital provision to care in the community; the pursuit of a primary health care team approach in a health centre; and, the deployment of the nurse in the family practitioner services. These were chosen as examples of innovative practice, with potential implications for the health manpower process.

CONCLUSION

This Chapter has outlined a methodology to investigate health manpower. As a guiding framework resort was made to Mejia's (1978) concept of the health manpower process. Exploration of its dimensions - planning, production and management - and their integration was argued to provide a fuller understanding of the state of manpower practices within a country's health services, as well as the potential for modification. This analysis must also extend to constraints, obstacles and facilitating factors. This leads on to a clarification and recognition of the political context surrounding manpower, in terms of policy formulation, implementation and evaluation.

A possible approach to the exploration of three areas in the manpower field was outlined: current manpower, supportive practices and future manpower requirements. Throughout, the importance and difficulty of finding out the 'true' state of affairs was expressed. Several strategies were suggested: identifying rationales behind planning decisions and documents; monitoring the implementation of plans; developing evaluative checklists and criteria against which current manpower practices can be judged; and challenging present positions, from a review of the current state through to an exploration of how a desired future health service together with desired manpower utilisation and deployment patterns (with implications for production and so on) can be achieved. The necessity of exploring the 'complete' manpower process, not just one or two of its dimensions, was stressed, along with mechanisms for their integration.

Finally, the methodology adopted in a one-year study of health manpower practices within the NHS in England and Wales was outlined. The study itself was set against the background of WHO's 'Health for All' strategy and its resultant manpower implications. While in the British study the primary focus lay on the planning and management dimensions of the health manpower process, production questions were also raised. In addition, mechanisms - both constraints and facilitators - for integrating these elements were elucidated. The approach concentrated on a review of the relevant literature, interviewing key actors, and preliminary attempts at generating criteria to evaluate manpower practices. The timescale of the project necessitated a foreshortening of its scope and breadth. While the major data collection was concentrated in 1984/5, the literature review has been continued, tracing manpower policy debates into 1986. The Chapters that follow present the findings of this study, from the contextual aspects of the British NHS, discussions of the manpower process within medical, nursing and allied health professions, survey data on manpower practices, case studies of manpower innovations in the primary health care arena, and a review of the issues of implementation and evaluation. It is to a discussion of the organisational context of the British NHS and its manpower that attention now turns.

Chapter 3

THE ORGANISATIONAL CONTEXT

This Chapter sets out to provide information on the
context in which the British study of health
manpower was undertaken. It begins by looking at
the current arrangements for planning services,
together with the identification of service
priorities and central guidance on manpower. It
then presents some brief comments on the
production of manpower, and outlines the nature
and composition of the workforce. More detail is
given for two key occupational groups, namely
physicians and nurses. Finally, attention turns to
the management dimension, identifying recent
initiatives of particular significance for the
development of the health manpower process.

PLANNING AND PRIORITIES

The history of health planning in Britain is a
relatively short one in that no formal planning
system existed before 1976. Prior to its
introduction health planning as a concept was
strongly advocated primarily because it was seen
as the means to overcome some of the inherent biases
in the British health care system (Crossman, 1972).
Two major distorting factors have been identified.
Firstly, there was an over-emphasis on hospital or
capital planning, a direct result of the publication
in the early 1960's of A Hospital Plan for England
and Wales (MoH, 1962). Secondly, the health care
network was split between hospital facilities, local
government health services, and family practitioner
services (which included general practitioners,
pharmacists, opticians and dentists), with each
dimension overseen by a separate administrative and
decision making body - a fragmentation which worked
to no-one's advantage (Rathwell, 1984). Any
planning done was not suprisingly largely unco-
ordinated and incremental, managers responding to

current situations and the decisions taken generally not forming part of any national or co-ordinated policy initiatives. The concentration on hospital buildings was accompanied by little, if any, regard for corresponding service and staff implications.

By the early 1970s this incremental approach to planning was seen by central policy makers as most unsatisfactory. What was needed was a more structured and rational approach to the management and development of health services. This led to the decision to adopt a rational, comprehensive model of health planning in Britain. Firstly, there was the growing awareness and interest in corporate management and the ideas associated with such a concept. Secondly, there was the general desire by central government for greater cost control within government departments, coupled with efforts by the Treasury to encourage these departments to present their financial forecasts in a more comprehensive and rigorous manner. Finally, there were the changes occurring in health care provision and delivery - development and expansion of high technology medicine and the costs associated with it - which highlighted the need for greater cost consciousness and consumer awareness in the NHS.

Thus, the creation and adoption of a formal planning system by the NHS was founded on the following precepts: a concern to overcome the incremental approach to planning characteristic of the 1960s and early 1970s; a desire to integrate and thereby improve the services for patients; and, a wish to introduce a concept of health planning which would be more reflective of the 'needs' of patients (DHSS, 1972; Rathwell, 1984). This philosophy of planning was embodied in the manual The NHS Planning System (DHSS, 1976a) which was distributed to all Health Authorities simultaneously when the corporate planning system was launched nationally in 1976. The formulation and implementation of the NHS planning system was accompanied by two major policy documents: Priorities for Health and Personal Social Services in England (DHSS, 1976b), which sought to re-orient the delivery of health care services through the identification of specific client groups considered to be particularly deserving of additional resources; and the other Sharing Resources for Health in England (DHSS, 1976c), which addressed the thorny issues of the way in which central resources were distributed among Health Authorities and offered a formal mechanism designed to achieve their more equitable distribution.

The Priorities document was a new departure for central policy makers, because it was the first time that an attempt had been made '... to establish rational and systematic priorities throughout the health and personal social services' (DHSS, 1976b, p.1). It was seen very much as the central or national strategy of health care objectives for the NHS in England, and encompassed two major thrusts. Firstly, it advocated the maintenance and where possible expansion of existing services. This philosophy was summarised in the following manner - 'to put people before buildings' (p.2). The second key feature of the document was its restatement of the importance of the role of primary health care which was coupled with the view that care within the community was potentially a 'better' way of meeting 'needs' (Chaplin, 1982). Particular groups were singled out for special attention (for example, the elderly, mentally ill, mental handicapped, and children) and specific targets (financial as well as service provision) were identified for each of these 'priority groups'.

The document, Sharing Resources for Health in England (similar documents were published for the Scottish, Welsh, and Northern Ireland health services) was concerned with the development of a method of resource distribution that was objective, equitable, and responsive to relative need (DHSS, 1976c). The formulae for allocating resources to Health Authorities were based on measures of relative need, and included such factors as population size and composition, morbidity, costs, and patient flows or mobility across administrative boundaries. The document was welcomed because of its attempt to re-direct the manner in which the financial resources available to the NHS were being allocated away from the 'cycle of creeping incremental privilege' towards the application of a method designed '... to determine logical bases for differential allocations of growth' (Chaplin, 1982, p.235).

These two policy documents were largely regarded as being separate and distinct rather than as an integrated package. This has led to a number of difficulties within the NHS. Although the Priorities document acknowledged the importance of tackling the problem of the geographical distribution of resources it attempted to respond to this shortcoming by stating that there was a need

'for a shift of resources towards those regions
and localities which historically have received
less funds per head of population than others,
and where standards of service have suffered
accordingly' (DHSS, 1976b, p.13).

Those responsible for the development of the
formulae for the allocation of resources
unfortunately took a more narrow position with
regard to the inextricable link between the
distribution and deployment when they declared that
'we have not regarded our remit as being concerned
with how the resources are deployed' (DHSS, 1976c,
p.8). Thus, the euphoria surrounding the
introduction of a formal planning system and these
two policy documents, which were essentially
promoting what might be considered as radical
changes for the NHS, was unlikely to last because of
the failure to integrate the concepts embodied
therein.

In consequence, the directional changes
identified have only now been partially achieved.
The NHS was quick to endorse the concept of
priority groups; this was widely reflected in the
multitude of strategic and operational plans that
have been produced since 1976 by Health Authorities.
However, the available evidence suggests that most
Health Authorities were less than enthusiatic about
implementing such policy changes (Rathwell and
Barnard, 1985). It is equally clear that
attempts to alter the pattern of resource allocation
have also had a mixed reception and correspondingly
have only had a limited impact (Bevan and Spencer,
1984). Commentators have attributed this lack of
concrescence between central policies and local
implementation to the dilemma of trying to impose a
national strategy whilst simultaneously allowing
local discretion. Insistence on a national
strategy, for example, could mean that in places
improvements may well be incompatible with local
circumstances. Further, if the strategy is
considered a desirable but non-binding level of
service, there is a risk that a continuing debate
over priorities will overshadow any meaningful
discussion of service improvements. To a large
extent this is precisely what has occurred (Rathwell
and Barnard, 1985).

The original concept of health planning based
on the twin details of rationality and
comprehensiveness was subsequently judged to be
'over-complicated and bureaucratic'; what was

required was a simpler planning system (DHSS, 1979a, p.18). The fact that there was some dissatisfaction with the planning process did not undermine the commitment of both the DHSS and the NHS to the discipline of planning, nor the belief that planning was still the most acceptable vehicle for determining and implementing national and local policies for health care. Nonetheless, the NHS planning system was duly amended and the system adopted placed considerable emphasis on strategic planning in the context of national policies and priorities (Health Circular HC(82)6 and HC(84)2). Current national initiatives in health care can be divided into two camps: priority groups and services; and community care. Each will be briefly discussed.

Publication of the booklet 'Care in Action' (DHSS, 1981a) reaffirmed the commitment 'to plan and develop services in the light of local needs and circumstances ... [having] regard to national policies and priorities' (p.i). The booklet re-emphasised the national priorities on the lines of earlier DHSS publications, and identified additional areas, namely: maternity services and neonatal care; primary care services; the care of young children at risk and the care and treatment of juvenile offenders (p.20); all in addition to the elderly, the mentally ill and handicapped.

The second policy thrust of the DHSS, embodied in the document 'Care in the Community' (DHSS, 1981b), argued for a 'shift in the balance of resources from hospital to the community services' (p.1). The rationale for such a policy was based on the view that 'there are many people in hospital who would not need to be there if appropriate community services are available' (ibid). It was envisaged that any initiatives designed to care for people in the community would of necessity involve very close liaison with the complementary local government departments of social services and housing. The document suggested that attempts to implement the policy of community care should in the first instance be confined to such groups as the elderly, the mentally ill and the mentally handicapped, because these are 'groups of people whose needs for care are most easily predictable' (p.13).

Within this context Health Authorities are now required to produce both strategic and operational plans, a process that occurs on two levels. Firstly, each District Health Authority (DHA) is delegated to prepare a strategic plan covering a 10 year planning period. In addition each DHA must also produce a short-term operational (two year) programme which outlines the steps that will be taken towards the implementation of national and local policies discussed in the strategic plan. The second level of activity occurs at the Regional Health Authority (RHA). Each RHA - of which there are 14 in England, but none in Scotland and Wales - is responsbile for preparing a Region-wide strategic plan which draws together the strategic plans from the DHAs within its boundary. However, prior to this each RHA must prepare and circulate to its DHAs an outline strategy which identifies those issues seen within the RHA as being of particular concern. This outline strategy is also submitted to the DHSS for approval. Once approved, the Regional outline strategy becomes the basis upon which each DHA prepares its strategic plan. Table 3.1 gives an indication of the relevant stages and the timescale within the strategic planning process.

As a final element in the planning process, each Regional strategic plan is submitted to the DHSS. In this way the Department is able to construct a composite picture of the degree of adherence to national policies and to identify any deviation from established targets. This so-called 'top-down bottom-up' approach to planning is justified on the grounds that

'it provides the opportunity for the Government's policies and priorities to be reconciled with available resources [whilst] it also enables health authorities to appraise systematically their own services and to influence the Government' (DHSS, 1981a, p.18).

Thus, through resource distribution and indications of national priorities the DHSS imposes its view on Regions, who then redraw such issues for their own context and set the boundaries for District plans. The DHA explores its own priorities and needs through planning teams and/or unit management groups, which are then channelled up the system. And so the cycle continues.

Table 3.1: NHS Planning System - Strategic Plans,
1985-94

Level	Tasks	Timescale
RHA	*to prepare outline strategy and send copy to DHSS	mid-May 1984
	*amend subject to DHSS comments and send outline strategy to DHAs	end May 1984
	*prepare Regional strategic plan incorporating DHA strategic plans and send to DHSS	end March 1985
	*send summary report to DHSS on main changes outlined in short term programme and on manpower targets	annually by end of March
DHA	*prepare 10 year strategic plan based upon Regional outline strategy	date to be agreed between DHA & RHA
	*prepare and submit to RHA and District short term programme including manpower targets	date to be agreed between DHA & RHA

Source: Health Circular HC(84)2

THE MANPOWER COMPONENT IN PLANNING

One of the major priorities of the planning system is manpower, in particular the co-ordination of manpower requirements with known service developments, and also the need to match service and manpower plans with available revenue (Table 3.2).

Table 3.2: Indications of National Guidance Related to Manpower

Plans should take full account of the manpower consequences of planned changes in service provision, of maintaining the present level and pattern of service, and of manpower shortages or mismatches. The Department will continue to provide information on the likely supply of those staff groups where there is a national dimension to planning.
The NHS Planning System HC(82)6 March 1982

As a step towards this, the Department is discussing with RHAs indicative figures which would achieve by 31 March 1984 a reduction of 0.75% to 1% in overall staff numbers from the total employed at 31 March 1983. Within that, posts other than doctors and dentists, nurses and midwives, and professional and technical are expected to reduce more sharply, by between 1.35% and 1.8%.

Health Authorities are expected to continue to seek ways of making more effective use of manpower resources and for ensuring that there is a service justification for every post created. In particular, no vacancy should be filled unless there is a clear case for its continuation. RHAs are asked to satisfy themselves that there are appropriate systems for this in DHAs and in the RHA-managed services. Progress towards targets will be monitored using the quarterly manpower counts and differences will be taken up with RHAs and discussed in the Regional review process.
Cash Limits and Manpower Targets for 1983-84 HC(83)16 August 1983

RHAs are expected to assess DHA programmes and satisfy themselves that they ... contain viable manpower targets consistent with the service objectives and the cash available and generally represent a good return on the investment of resources.

The manpower targets exercise in 1983 was a necessary response to a failure by Health Authorities to secure adequate manpower planning and control .... Manpower control should become an explicit feature of the system for producing and approving short term programmes. Ministers will continue for the time being to monitor manpower carefully in order to be satisfied that the proposed system is working smoothly.... Any growth in staff numbers should continue the existing trends of concentration on those groups who deliver services direct to patients. Any increase in staff numbers over the agreed baseline must be explained by reference to improvements in service which cannot be achieved by improvements in performance or redeployment from elsewhere.
Resource Distribution for 1984-85, Service Priorities, Manpower and Planning HC(84)2 January 1984

More effective monitoring of NHS manpower numbers has been introduced: manpower limits have been settled, complementing authorities' cash limits.
Implementation of the NHS Management Inquiry Report HC(84)13 June 1984

The manpower indicators are not entirely compatible with the indicators for clinical activity, which are specialty specific, nor with financial indicators which are hospital specific. Particular problems have been experienced in the collection and validation of data for manpower indicators, particularly those affected by the distribution of nurse learners, and so these performance indicators (PIs) should be treated with still greater caution than other PIs.
Performance Indicators: An Introductory Guide for Users, DHSS 1983a

---

So for example in 1982 the DHSS (HC(82)14) spelt out its requirements for annual planning programmes to include manpower targets, thus ensuring that such targets reflected revenue assumptions. The stated concern was deploying manpower 'to the maximum effect in the interests of patient care'. This was followed up in early 1983 with a communication which stated that any increase in manpower must result in increases in the volume

or quality of services (HC(83)4). Few could
disagree with this emphasis, but an additional
circular produced later in that year made plain that
its prime motivation was the control of costs and
manpower, rather than a concern with effectiveness
and patient care (HC(83)16). 'Firm' manpower
targets, involving manpower 'control' were outlined:
a 0.75 to 1% reduction in overall numbers, but for
posts other than doctor, dentist, nurse and midwife,
and professional and technical, a sharper reduction
of 1.35 to 1.8% was envisaged. Furthermore, for
every vacancy created, 'no vacancy should be filled
unless there is a clear case for its (the post's)
continuation' (ibid).

The recent planning guidance from the DHSS
states that 'in the future manpower control should
become an explicit feature of the system' (HC(84)2).
Within this planning philosophy it is acknowledged
that manpower changes will be slower to achieve than
developments in services and revenue commitments,
and 'any growth in staff numbers should continue
existing trends of concentration on those groups who
deliver services direct to patients' (ibid). In
fact, the guidance is emphatic that

> 'any increase in staff numbers over the agreed
> baseline must be explained by reference to
> improvements in services which cannot be
> achieved by improvements in performance or
> redeployment' (ibid).

The difficulty with guidance such as this is that,
whilst transferring the onus onto DHAs for manpower
targets and planning, it fails to offer any
mechanism or procedure for DHAs to follow when
attempting to incorporate this policy into their
strategic plans. The consequences for the health
manpower process of such vague policy making,
coupled with the current climate concerned with
costs, efficiency and central control are discussed
below.

THE PRODUCTION OF MANPOWER AND SIZE OF THE WORKFORCE

The NHS is the largest single employer in Britain.
It employs over 1 million people whose wages and
salaries account for approximately 70% of total
health care expenditure. The following table (Table
3.3) gives a broad indication of the numbers of
staff employed in the NHS.

Such figures do not show the numbers employed

Table 3.3: NHS Staff and Practitioners - United Kingdom, September 30, 1983 (whole time equivalents, thousands)

	ENGLAND	SCOTLAND	WALES	N. IRELAND	TOTAL	%
Medical and Dental	38.7	6.1	2.4	1.7	48.9	4.5
Nursing and Midwifery	393.7	62.3	26.0	18.9	500.9	45.7
Professional/Technical	68.7	9.2	4.2	2.5	84.6	7.7
Works/Maintenance	26.8	3.8	2.1	1.2	33.9	3.1
Administrative/Clerical	110.0	14.1	6.5	4.8	135.4	12.4
Ambulance Personnel	18.4	1.7	1.4	0.6	22.1	2.0
Ancillary	166.2	27.0	11.6	8.6	213.4	19.5
General Medical Practitioners	25.3	3.5	1.5	0.9	31.2	2.8
General Dental Practitioners	13.7	1.4	0.7	0.4	16.2	1.5
Other Practitioners	8.1	0.7	0.5	0.1	9.4	0.9
Overall Total	869.6	129.8	56.9	39.7	1095.9	100.1

Source: Central Statistical Office, 1985, Table 4.12 adapted.

37

in the private health sector. However, it is not
the size or actual numbers of those working in the
private health sector which is of particular
importance, but rather that both health sectors,
public and private, are competing for a finite pool
of staff. It is finite because the number of
training places are controlled outwith the health
sectors and bears little or no relation to the
ability of each sector to absorb or employ such
trained staff. Thus arrangements for education and
training of staff necessary for providing health
care services are undertaken separately from the
processes applied to determining the sorts of staff
and their appropriate skills required by the health
sector.

A critical factor affecting the supply of
qualified manpower is the number of training places
available for the various staff groups, the exact
control over number, and content of education and
training varying extensively. The role of agencies
outside the NHS in determining health manpower is
considerable, especially in those instances where
the professional associations operate simultaneously
as trade unions representing the profession. Their
influence is directed at the numbers in which
manpower is produced, the roles for which they
train and subsequently adopt, and in some cases
the workload which they are expected to undertake.

The continuum shown in Figure 3.1 illustrates
the determinants of the number of training places
available in various occupations in the British
health sector. These are, of course, not the sole
determinants, since the number trained will normally
be less than the number of places, due to such
factors as failure and drop-out rates. The left-
hand extreme of the continuum illustrates the groups
of staff who are trained 'on the job' and where the
Health Authority is the sole determining agency.
Movement towards the right-hand end of the continuum
indicates an increase in the number of institutions
involved. For each of the groups of staff plotted,
a list of agencies involved is set out. For example
for nursing, schools are located at the District
level; the tutors and the students are Health
Authority employees. Other institutions involved are
the relevant Regional Nurse Training Committee
(RNTC), which funds the salaries of teaching and
support staff, as well as capital resources, and the
English National Board for Nursing, Midwifery and

Figure 3·1 A Model of Training Places [a]

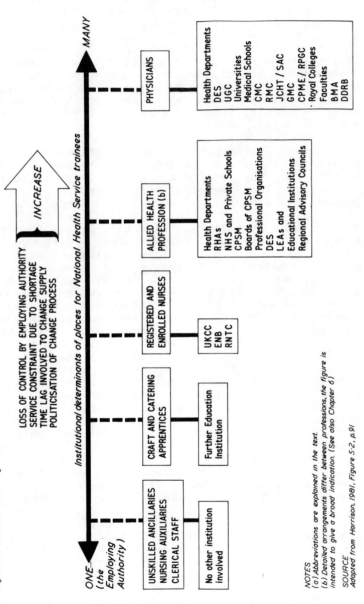

LOSS OF CONTROL BY EMPLOYING AUTHORITY
SERVICE CONSTRAINT DUE TO SHORTAGE
TIME LAG INVOLVED IN CHANGE SUPPLY
POLITICISATION OF CHANGE PROCESS

INCREASE

ONE — (the Employing Authority)

Institutional determinants of places for National Health Service trainees

MANY

UNSKILLED ANCILLARIES NURSING AUXILIARIES CLERICAL STAFF	CRAFT AND CATERING APPRENTICES	REGISTERED AND ENROLLED NURSES	ALLIED HEALTH PROFESSION (b)	PHYSICIANS
No other institution involved	Further Education Institution	UKCC ENB RNTC	Health Departments RHAs NHS and Private Schools CPSM Boards of CPSM Professional Organisations DES LEAs and Educational Institutions Regional Advisory Councils	Health Departments DES UGC Universities Medical Schools CMC RMC JCHT / SAC GMC CPME / RPGC Royal Colleges Faculties BMA DDRB

NOTES
(a) Abbreviations are explained in the text.
(b) Detailed arrangements differ between professions, the figure is
intended to give a broad indication. (See also Chapter 6)

SOURCE
Adapted from Harrison, 1981, Figure 5·2, p.91

39

Health Visiting (ENB) which sets syllabi and standards and 'licenses' schools and the hospitals to which students are attached for practical training. There are also Boards for Wales, Scotland and Northern Ireland.

Further to the right come the allied health professionals. For example, local education authorities (LEAs) are involved in providing grants to students of schools not located in hospitals, whilst central Health Departments provide grants to other students. LEAs administer the former type of school, whilst Regional Health Authorities provide funds for the latter.

Finally, the production of physicians, located towards the extreme right of the continuum, are subject to the influence of a large number of agencies. The number of medical undergraduates is controlled somewhat indirectly; funds originate from the Department of Education and Science (DES), and are routed through the University Grants Committee (UGC) to individual universities. Although each university is normally free to allocate resources between academic departments as it sees fit, UGC policies are in practice adhered to. In the case of medicine the relevant policy emanates from the DHSS. Basic standards for medical qualifications are determined by the General Medical Council (GMC) with whom practicing doctors must register. Institutions involved in postgraduate medical education and qualification have to be added to the list. The Central and Regional Manpower Committees (CMCs, RMCs) and RHAs are involved in the allocation of vacancies to specific specialties and locations, whereas the Royal Colleges and Faculties are able to accredit posts as adequate for training in particular specialties. Joint Committees on Higher Training (JCHTs) and their Specialty Advisory Committees (SACs) are responsible for the accreditation of Senior Registrars as suitable for promotion to Consultant, whilst postgraduate medical education is co-ordinated by Councils for Postgraduate Medical Education (CPMEs) and Regional Postgraduate Medical Education Committees (RPGCs). Finally, the activities of institutions involved in formal collective bargaining, the British Medical Association (BMA) and the Review Body on Doctors' and Dentists' Remuneration (DDRB), need to be included since the format of doctors' contracts and distribution of relative earnings in the profession will affect the numbers and roles of practitioners.

It is thus apparent that there is at least a

potential divergence between the production and planning dimension, over numbers produced, curricula and the like, with consequences for the management dimension of the manpower process, over roles and utilisation patterns. What though are the constituent sizes of the major occupational groups, namely doctors and nurses, and basic education and training arrangements?

Looking first of all at the medical workforce, the intake to British medical schools stood at 3,951 in 1983. The undergraduate course is divided into pre-clinical and clinical years, and generally lasts for 5 years. After successful completion of these studies the medical graduate undertakes a pre-registration year - typically in hospital - in order to qualify fully with the General Medical Council. At this juncture, the career paths for hospital consultants, general practitioners (GPs) and those pursuing community medicine diverge. Three main grades are recognised:

1 autonomous career grades: hospital consultant, general practitioner, and community physician;

2 postgraduate training grades: junior doctors in hospital - Senior Registrar, Senior House Officer (SHO), Pre- and Post-Registration House Officer (HO), and trainee GP;

3 non-training grades: Clinical Assistant, Hospital Practitioner, Senior House Medical Officer, and Associate Specialist (formerly Medical Assistant).

Consultants alone exercise full clinical autonomy in the delivery of health care in hospitals. They also supervise the training of junior doctors, and additionally, oversee the clinical activities of those in the non-training grades.

The figures contained in Table 3.4 provide a picture of the NHS medical workforce in September 1984 with a breakdown by grade. While this records the actual numbers in each hospital grade, all other medical staff are given as whole-time equivalents (WTEs). In the hospital service the WTE translates to 42,794 doctors overall, with 14,794 consultants, 24,827 juniors and 3,225 in the non-training grades (National Audit Office, 1985a, p.12). Part-time engagements are most prevalent among the non-training grades as all Hospital Practitioners and

42

Table 3.4: The Medical Career Structure and Numbers, 30 September 1984 for Great Britain

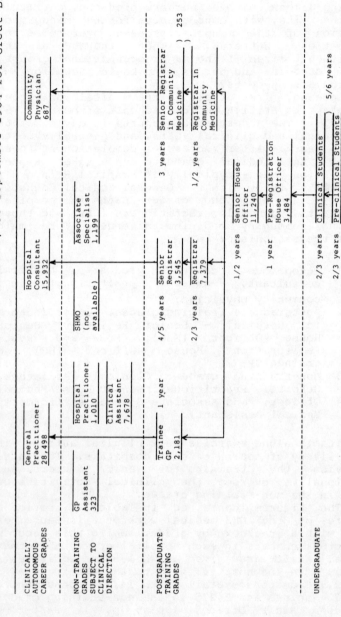

Source: National Audit Office, 1985a, pp.25-26, adapted.
Note: Figures are for September 1984, Great Britain. Figures for the hospital grades are actual staff numbers
        not whole time equivalents.

nearly all Clinical Assistants are also Principals in general practice.

The length of time spent in postgraduate training before becoming a hospital consultant has usually been between seven and eleven years with considerable variation across specialisms. Indeed, the hospital career structure has become much more complex in recent years with more than one hundred listed medical and dental specialties and sub-specialties.

While still a small minority of the dental profession as a whole, the hospital dental services have grown considerably since 1948. There are currently over 400 consultants in the dental specialties with the commensurate junior 'tail'. This compares with a total stock of dentists in 1982 of some 22,500 (DHSS, 1983b). In 1983 766 entered dental schools in England and Wales. In the organisation across grades the career structure of dental practitioners almost exactly mirrors that of their medical counterparts.

As for the nursing workforce, nursing staff constitute almost one half of NHS employees. Their wages comprise 45% of the total wage bill and a third of the total revenue expenditure. The figures for WTEs of nursing and midwifery staff in 1983 are included in Table 3.5. The category 'nurse' is the subject of much dispute and not a little bitterness. Official Health Department returns for nurse staffing levels employ 'nurse' as a general umbrella term to include qualified persons, learners, and more contentiously, unqualified staff - nursing auxiliaries and aides. A small number of agency nursing and midwifery staff can be added to these totals. Hospital staff form the largest single group but important primary and community personnel - most notably, district nurses, those working in general practice, and health visitors - are also included.

The nursing workforce has long demonstrated high internal differentiation in skills and specialisation, and these have increased over the life of the NHS. A fundamental division exists between qualified nursing staff and unqualified nursing auxiliaries. The former include state registered nurses (SRNs) who have undergone a three year training course, and state enrolled nurses (SENs) who have taken a two year qualification. State registration as midwife, district nurse or health visitor requires successful completion of further appropriate professional training and

43

Table 3.5: Nursing and Midwifery Staff in Great Britain, 30 September 1983

Status	England 1983	Wales 1983	Scotland 1983	Great Britain 1983	% of Total
Total	394,685	25,981	62,396	483,062[1]	100
Qualified	223,612	14,974	32,232	270,818	56
Registered	153,594	9,808	21,910	185,312	38
Enrolled	70,018	5,166	10,322	85,506	18
Learners[2]	78,856	4,131	12,402	95,389	20
Unqualified[3]	92,217	6,876	17,762	116,855	24

Source: National Audit Office, 1985b, p.23, adapted.

Notes: [1] Excludes agency nursing and midwifery staff (approximately 2,500 at 30 September 1983). The total WTE figures including agency nursing staff for 1983 are 417,000 and 486,000 the majority of agency nurses are employed in England; the numbers of Scotland and Wales are marginal.

[2] Includes health visitor and district nurse students, student midwives and post-basic hospital nursing students.

[3] Includes nursing cadets.

examination. The category of unqualified staff covers those such as nursing auxiliaries, nursery nurses and blood attendants who may well have undergone a period of training for their work but who have not completed a course of professional education. As the divide between qualified and unqualified staff is crucial so too the distinction between registered and enrolled nurses separates off the former who alone are eligible for promotion through the nursing grade hierarchy. This ranges from initial appointment as a Staff Nurse through: (i) Nursing Sister/Charge Nurse who has charge of a ward and its nursing staff; (ii) Senior Nurse who may operate in a 'staff support' or a 'clinical-managerial' function; (iii) Director of Nursing Services (DNS) who manages a unit's nursing services and related budget in conjunction with administrative and medical staff; (iv) District or Chief Nursing Officer and (v) Regional Nursing Officer. These last two act in an advisory capacity to their respective Health Authorities under current arangements for general management in the NHS.

A further differentiation of nursing staff is provided by area of specialisation. Enrolled nurses include those with general, mental nursing or mentally handicapped qualifications. Registered staff include: general, mental, mental handicapped, and sick children's nurses, as well as district nurses, midwives and health visitors. All of these nurses are registered with the United Kingdom Central Council for Nursing, Midwifery and Health Visiting (UKCC) which took over previous statutory and training board functions for these groups in 1983. The majority of nursing staff are employed in hospitals. Community nursing services are provided by community midwives, psychiatric and mental handicap nurses, district nurses, health visitors, and school nurses. These services are supplemented by nurses employed by general practitioners.

THE MANAGEMENT DIMENSION

Since 1974 the NHS has undergone two major organisational changes, both conceived and implemented in the name of efficiency. The first, in 1982, saw the abolition of the Area tier of management and the banishment of consensus management on the grounds that such a management structure created indecision and excessive

bureaucracy. The recipe for remedying this
situation was to bring the decision-making process
as close to the local community as possible and
therefore give those in the community as well as
the providers of service the opportunity to
participate in policy-making (DHSS, 1979a).

Shortly after the transition from a three-
(Region, Area, District) to a two-tiered
administrative (Region, District) structure the
Secretary of State for Health and Social Services
established the National Health Service Management
Inquiry to

'review current initiatives to improve the
efficiency of the health service, and to advise
on the management action needed to secure the
best value for money and the best possible
service to patients' (DHSS, 1983c).

The 'Griffiths Report' contained many
recommendations such as the creation of supervisory
and management boards within the DHSS; greater
involvement of clinicians in management; the
encouragement of better performance through the use
of incentives and/or sanctions; and improvements in
management techniques. However, the recommendation
to establish general managers at each level of NHS
management has become the most profound and
contentious issue arising out of the Inquiry.
Simply put, the role of the General Manager, as a
replacement for the team approach evident in the
days of consensus management, was to ensure that
responsibility and accountability for decision-
making rested in one, named, individual.

Allied to the introduction of general
management was the desire of the DHSS to strengthen
the accountability procedure between itself and the
semi-autonomous Health Authorities. This was
accomplished by establishing an Annual Review
Process (ARP) whereby each Health Authority, in
effect, had to report to the DHSS on the progress
achieved over the ensuing year. The process begins
with the DHSS issuing specific targets or objectives
in accordance with established national policies or
priorities to Regional Health Authorities to achieve
over the coming year; at the end of the year the
RHAs are held accountable for their progress.
Failure to achieve these pre-determined policies or
objectives is carefully scrutinised with the
implicit threat that non-achievement without just

cause could have serious implications especially as the DHSS is responsible for the allocation of resources to the RHAs. RHAs in turn make similar demands on the Health Districts within their boundaries. This too carries a potential threat as RHAs have the responsibility for the allocation of financial resources to the Districts.

Almost contemporaneously, a set of performance indicators (PIs) were introduced by the DHSS to aid Health Authorities in assessing the service they provided, and particularly its cost. An initial range of indicators was prepared; these included activities such as clinical, manpower, financial, laundry, accident and emergency, ambulance, and estate management (DHSS, 1983a). PIs were seen not only as a supplement to existing management information, but also as a mechanism for assisting managers in identifying those services which warrant examination and investigation. Such PIs were derived from existing nationally available data. This focus is however an inherent weakness because such data are overwhelmingly activity-based, so that the emphasis is slanted towards the efficient use of resources (activity generated per unit of resource), and is less concerned with effectiveness of care (impact of the service on the population). Nonetheless, they provide a starting point for management in pursuit of their monitoring and evaluative responsibilities. The 1981 based set of PIs has been substantially revamped to take account of earlier criticisms, and also to introduce additional indicators. The 1983 and 1984 based indicators bear little resemblance to their early cousins.

There is also the issue of the information base for health manpower planning. As Cree (1981) has outlined, the development of a computer-based, standard (in terms of definitions and items collected), and accessible data base has a high priority. Currently, information on the stock of manpower is reasonably accessible through the use of the standard manpower planning and personnel information system (STAMP), a computer based system that draws on existing payroll records. Unfortunately, little or no information is available from the STAMP system on the flows between grades, qualifications possessed or career histories. Sample surveys must be undertaken in order to fill in this gap (for example, Long et al, 1983). Furthermore, a paucity of information exists on the potential supply of manpower. Current initiatives from the Korner review of information (Korner, 1984) and DHSS advice to Health Authorities (HC(84)10) will help in providing a minimum data set but one which only relates to manpower stock characteristics. National and Regional policy on computer developments, District access to them, and the use of micro-computers, is a further issue of relevance because it opens up the possibility whereby each DHA may opt to develop its own local manpower database which would be specifically tailored to local requirements, rather than rely on the national system and its known inconsistencies. It is worth noting that this is an area which is experiencing rapid changes with new databases and suites to analyse the data being developed (for example, the Manpower Management System).

A final managerial initiative in the manpower arena relates to the formulation of an advisory group on manpower. In 1976, the DHSS established a joint DHSS/NHS forum for the exploration of manpower planning issues, the Joint Manpower Planning and Information Working Group, known as MAPLIN (Petch, 1981). The development of STAMP and various reports on particular manpower problems arose from such meetings, the most notable being the guide to local manpower planning entitled <u>Managing the Manpower Future</u> (MAPLIN 1981). Whilst MAPLIN has since been disbanded, a new central group has been formed (the Manpower Planning Advisory Group) comprising NHS Regional Chief Officers from nursing, medicine, finance, works, personnel and administration. In 1986, its chairperson became the Personnel Director of the Management Board of the NHS. Its brief is to identify key issues in NHS manpower planning where attention needs to be focussed, such as supply and demand issues for particular professions, the manpower input to strategic plans, the investment in training and geographical imbalances in the output from training establishments.

CONCLUSION

Despite the commonplace acceptance that the marriage between manpower and service planning, production and management is a necessity, considerable progress remains to be made. Several difficulties need to be resolved. Firstly, there is the professionalisation of manpower within each occupational group, playing a major role in determining not only how many of each particular group there should be, but also the training, education, qualifications and experience they should possess. This issue is explored more fully within later Chapters. A second and related factor concerns the mismatch between supply and demand. The role of the professional associations such as the British Medical Association and Royal Colleges for doctors, and the RCN, National Boards and the UKCC for nurses is crucial, since it is largely these bodies who determine, if not the actual numbers to be trained, what the curricula should contain and what the eligibility criteria should be. Thus one encounters the situation of the supply of certain groups of manpower being out of synchronisation with service requirements.

A third complicating feature is the distortion that central policy directives on manpower create within the service planning process. For example, the National Health Service Management Board recently amended manpower targets for the NHS with the net result that five of the fourteen RHAs had to operate with fewer staff than they asked for (DHSS, 1985a). It is the DHSS who limits the number of people by category of manpower to be employed by each Region, and by implication within each DHA, thus reducing scope for local initiatives on the size and mix of manpower necessary to achieve local service objectives. As Day and Klein (1985) so succinctly put it; 'the Regions may propose but it is the DHSS that disposes' (p.1676).

A fourth and final issue concerns the disparity between the way resources are allocated to the NHS and the procedure for service planning. Because resource allocation is undertaken separately from the planning process it is not unusual for plans to be produced on rather uncertain financial assumptions. This uncertainty spills over into the manpower element of such plans, since it is often the availability of manpower which dictates the sort of services to be provided and not, as is commonly held, the other way round.

The changes in organisation structure (for planning and management) together with the greater control being exercised by the centre in the NHS at present highlight an organisation in flux. It remains to be seen in what ways the introduction of general management and the Annual Review Process encourage closer attention to the apparent incongruence of manpower planning, production and management. Currently, issues of efficiency (themselves activity-focused, and with little concern for quality or consumer satisfaction) and cost control predominate (Long and Harrison, 1985).

The Organisational Context

The potential for the use of such organisational processes for the introduction of positive stimuli to the health manpower process obviously exists: for example, a move towards integrating manpower production with planning, and planning with management practice; and a move towards PHC and multidisciplinary team working. But so far this is a dormant potential.

Chapter 4

MEDICAL MANPOWER

An impending crisis in the management of medical
staff has been a recurring theme in debates about
the 'state of the NHS'. At first sight this seems
paradoxical. After all, some 90% of active
registered physicians undertake work in the NHS, and
nearly all postgraduate training is located in NHS
hospitals. Furthermore, it has been claimed in one
authoritative text on the health services in Britain
that, '(i)n the field of manpower planning, the most
comprehensive arrangements within the NHS are those
relating to doctors and dentists' (Chaplin, 1982,
p.373). Yet professional, Health Authority and
governmental reviews of current practices have
consistently documented quite fundamental
shortcomings. While all sectors are now agreed on
the necessity to improve the health manpower
process, they are often at odds over the closer
details of the central problems and the
appropriateness of various policy options.

This Chapter sets out to identify and explore
the significant issues in medical manpower planning,
with special reference to hospital staff. General
medical and dental services (General Practitioners
and General Dental Practitioners) are dealt with in
more detail in Chapter Eight. The discussion
concentrates on the current state of the art, but
also focusses on those aspects which constrain the
formulation and implementation of manpower plans for
physicians.

PLANNING: MEDICAL STOCKS AND FLOWS

Any discussion of medical manpower must acknowledge
at the outset its inherent difficulties and
complexity: 'the reports of the past are milestones
on the hard road towards understanding' (Parkhouse,
1979, p.1). A comparison of early and current
excursions into medical manpower forecasting

demonstrates that considerable effort has been invested in the improvement of techniques and data in the estimation of supply and demand for staff. The Goodenough Report of 1944 argued that with the inception of the NHS more doctors would be required, and that there should therefore be an increase in the annual intake to British medical schools. Their calculations focussed on basic stocks and flows but were much hampered by the paucity of available data. They estimated that the existing intake of medical students would have to increase from around 2,000 to 2,500 in order to exceed the 50,000 stock of doctors by the early 1950s, although thereafter medical school recruitment might be reduced significantly.

Changing perspectives on the imbalance between demand for and supply of medical staff have been an enduring feature of the post-war years. The Willink Report of 1957 supported growing fears in the profession that a surplus of physicians was imminent. It recommended a 10% reduction in the number of new medical students as soon as practicable. For the most part the report's analysis concentrated on supply side factors; its demand estimates did not extend beyond doctor-to-population ratios. The lack of an adequate data base was acknowledged, and so its long term forecasts were regarded as highly speculative. The next few years cruelly exposed these weaknesses. Both the hospital services and population grew faster than anticipated. On the supply side the estimates of migration patterns grossly miscalculated the extent of immigration among foreign trained, mostly junior, doctors.

A series of critical reviews in the 1960s from a variety of sources encouraged the government to restore the 10% cut in student intake and to increase it by a further 15% to about 2,400. Even this expansion was overshadowed by fresh proposals in an interim report from the Royal Commission on Medical Education (Todd Report, 1968). This advocated a doubling in recruitment to medical schools to 4,700 in 1980 and 5,000 by 1985. The rationale underlying these recommendations incorporated both evidence of changing supply-side trends, as well as suggested improvements in the doctor-to-population ratios. For its part, the government set a target intake of 4,080 for the late 1970s, and although this has not yet been achieved because of expenditure constraints (in 1983 it stood at 3,951), it remains an official objective (DHSS, 1985a).

However, unease has resurfaced in the medical profession about an over-production of doctors - especially in the hospital services. Cut-backs in the medical school intake have been widely advocated. This is amply demonstrated in evidence from various medical organisations to the House of Commons Social Services Select Committee (Short Report, 1981; and 1985a) and has been consistently argued by the British Medical Association (Bolt, 1983).

Over the post-war years the central Health Departments have endeavoured to enhance the data, assumptions and techniques for projecting medical supply and demand. Especial interest has focussed on moving away from periodic, single estimate forecasts that took too little account of available resources towards: sensitivity analysis that allowed a range in the main assumptions and their likely effects; regular up-dating of the data base and continuous monitoring of the policy impact; and greater attention to financial constraints on the NHS (Maynard and Walker, 1977; Parkhouse, 1979).

The discussion paper entitled Medical Manpower - The Next Twenty Years (DHSS, 1978) set out the background to official thinking on medical forecasting. The emphasis on regular reviews of the situation has been accepted - with reports from the Medical Manpower Steering Group (DHSS, 1980a) and the Advisory Committee on Medical Manpower Planning (ACMMP) (DHSS, 1985a). As a consequence, the assumptions on which demand for and the supply of physicians are estimated have been spelt out, while detailed statistical information has also been provided.

Supply

It is evident from these inquiries that the central concepts on which manpower plans have been built have been subject to reformulation. The ACMMP report described supply and demand as 'both terms of art' (p.3). The former has been consistently viewed as encompassing those physicians in or actively seeking medical employment, as well as the level of intake to medical schools. A range of key supply side factors was elaborated: the size of the medical school intake; medical school wastage rates; emigration and immigration patterns; and changing physician activity rates, stemming especially from the increased proportion of females in medicine, and the trend toward earlier retirement among doctors (DHSS, 1978).

The pre-eminent issue for the medical profession has been the level of the medical school intake. It is noticeable that medical manpower planning has been slow to take up issues of the maldistribution of physicians - geographically, as well as across specialisms and between hospital and general medical sectors. As the ACMMP report acknowledges this means that even its projections are not easily disaggregated although it was not a central aim to 'predict exactly where the stock of doctors will be working in 20 years' time' (DHSS, 1985a, p.25). Efforts to encourage physicians to practice in poorly endowed areas as well as in shortage specialties have met with varying success. The trend since the early 1970s has been for the worst of the geographical disparities between RHAs to diminish although wide differences remain. The DHSS also claims that the distribution across specialisms has improved over the last decade. Specific problems nevertheless persist at the consultant level - most notably in geriatrics and mental illness which have been priority service care groups since the mid 1970s (National Audit Office, 1985a, p.9), although such shortages are being eliminated in the training grades (House of Commons, 1985a).

Changing migration patterns have further complicated the forecasting of doctor numbers. Particular attention has been directed to the growth in the proportion of overseas trained physicians in the NHS. Currently, about one third of hospital doctors (and more of juniors) and one fifth of general practitioners (GPs) qualified outside the British Isles. Migration trends and policies continue to be in a state of flux. A further source of foreign graduates has been added with entry to the EEC, although domestic legislation (Medical Act, 1978) has curbed immigration of physicians, while emigration opportunities to North America and Australia in particular have become more restricted.

Overseas doctors have for the most part been utilised as a reserve from which to draw junior hospital staff, and there has been much criticism of their lack of training and career prospects. In recent manpower forecasts these migration flows have been accorded more prominence, not least because any substantial expansion of British graduates within the junior doctor categories threatens a serious log jam in promotion prospects. Control of medical immigrants does at the same time provide a more immediate impact on doctor supply than restrictions on the medical school intake. In March 1985 the Secretary of State for Social Services announced new immigration rules designed to reduce the flow of foreign doctors into the NHS, whether seeking postgraduate training in hospital posts or employment as general practitioners. With the full support of the BMA, it was claimed that the UK has become self-sufficient in its supply of doctors and dentists (British Medical Journal, 6 April 1985, p.1087).

Unlike most other prestigious professional groups, medicine has taken steps to encourage female recruitment in recent years and the current medical school intake is now close to its parity target. Manpower planners have presumed that this trend will have consequences for the overall activity and participation rates of physicians. All of the latest DHSS calculations attempt to take these into account (DHSS, 1978; DHSS, 1985a). As with overseas doctors, pressure has been exerted by female practitioners to ensure a more equitable distribution of hospital posts across both grades and specialties. In addition, there has been much female lobbying for greater opportunities for part-time training and career positions.

The search for more accurate projections of the main elements in labour supply to medicine continues unabated (DHSS, 1985a). With continuing uncertainties and disagreements about the assumptions and estimates of supply trends, the main protagonists have experienced considerable difficulties in reaching agreement on the most apposite supply side policies for manpower plans. The professional interpretation of the 'manpower crisis' in the 1980s concentrates on the spectre of medical unemployment and the dislocation of the career structure with its associated waste of investment and human resources. The DHSS scenario as outlined in Medical Manpower (DHSS, 1978) was more sanguine about these medical fears. It did accept that problems might well arise because 'demands to use the available doctors would pre-empt resources and distort priorities' (p.36), but it did not forsee significant medical unemployment.

Demand

Current 'demand' estimates have been greatly swayed by pressure from the Health Departments for more realism in manpower planning. Medical Manpower

spelled out a definition of medical 'need' in terms
of the financial resources available to the NHS. It
offered as working assumptions that: the gross
national product (GNP) would continue to rise by
2.5% per year; the proportion of GNP devoted to
health care would not fall; the real growth in
health care resources would amount to 1.5%; and
expenditure on doctors would hold steady as a
proportion of the overall NHS budget (pp.11-13). In
the ACMMP report the reconstitution of demand in
narrow economic terms is well-nigh completed:

> 'The "demand" for doctors is the number of
> opportunities available for active work in
> medicine, that is the number of funded places
> available in health authorities, universities,
> other public bodies and the private sector,
> plus the number of opportunities in general
> medical practice. This is a rather different
> concept from the notion of the total underlying
> 'need' for medical care, or indeed from the
> total demands placed by individuals on the
> health services; such measures of demand may or
> may not equate with what is affordable ....
> Our concept of demand is therefore similar to
> the economist's notion of "effective demand" –
> that is, the number of doctors which our
> society, with given resources and preferences
> for spending those resources, will choose to
> employ if they are available' (DHSS, 1985a,
> pp.3-4).

At the same time the DHSS has reduced the long term
resource assumptions for health planning to around
a half per cent per year over the next ten years.
This still leaves considerable uncertainties
for manpower planning. Not least the correlation
between growth in resources and in manpower employed
is problematic: for example, the differential
resource assumptions across RHAs. This calculation
is rendered even more complex in the light of
central priorities to improve the availability of
medical care in several specialisms and to increase
the proportion of staff in the career grades.
Further resources for 'front line staff' could be
generated by Health Authorities if they reduce the
cost of existing services or if 'at the margin' they
'choose to substitute other staff or resources for
doctors in expanding their services' (p.22).
The situation in the general medical services
is not thought to pose the same problems. Growth in

the numbers of GPs is not so determined by the availability of financial resources, but rather by the supply of medical practitioners, and the demand for partners by existing GPs. Simple extrapolation of past trends in the demand for general medical services suggests a 2% annual growth that would reduce the average list size to something close to the current BMA target of 1,700 by the early 1990s. The ACMMP report (DHSS, 1985a) sees little prospect of that expansion being maintained, and emphasises that the growth in GP numbers is closely dependent on the demands for doctors in the hospital and community services, and to a lesser extent in private medicine.

This reformulation of demand for doctors is reinforced by the ACMMP report's generally dismissive comments on the alternative approaches highlighted as recently as the Medical Manpower document (DHSS, 1978). The extrapolation of rising trends in the doctor-to-patient quotient, and the analysis of manpower plans in Regional strategic plans are both regarded as flawed. Attempts to elaborate 'objective' measures of the need for medical services seemed to bear little fruit. Manpower forecasts were also confounded by the difficulties in arriving at informed projections of the impact on medical demand of: demographic factors; changes in medical practice; and improvements in the services provided. Indeed, closer inspection of the extent to which existing medical needs are unfulfilled in such areas as services for the elderly, mentally ill, obstetrics and gynaecology has produced conclusions which are largely unpalatable for the national Health Departments which wish to regard current medical manpower numbers and care as generally satisfactory (DHSS, 1980a).

Contributions from the medical community have emphasised the lack of resources facing the NHS, although it has been far from united in its preferred method of calculating manpower needs. The Todd Report of 1968 followed the generally favoured approach of linking demand to population growth, although more recently attention has been re-directed to particular groups who are felt to represent a higher call on medical resources - such as the elderly (Bolt, 1983). Typically, the demand for geriatricians is set in population terms - presently 3 consultants per 200,000 people. Another preoccupation in professional discussions is the impact on demand for physicians which stems from the development of new specialisms, knowledge and practices. Medical unity is therefore under constant threat as existing and new specialisms argue for a larger, or their own, slice of the NHS cake. Invariably the demand calculations return to a doctor-to-population ratio.

This is equally true of arguments that there should be a reduction in regional inequalities in health care, which are usually couched in terms of the less well-endowed Regions on the basis of doctor-to-population ratios being brought up to some higher standard. These claims are made both for the hospital and the general medical services. In the latter, the objective of lowering the list size has been almost the sole criterion of manpower forecasting, although the Royal College of General Practitioners has argued that future needs in general practice are difficult to calculate without detailed studies of the effectiveness of different types of care (Short Report, Vol. II, 1981, pp.297-310). Such an attitude remains the exception although the profession clearly feels that it is under increasing pressure to think firstly, in terms of 'how many doctors can we afford?' rather than 'how many doctors do we need?', and secondly, in terms of the relative costs and contribution of different skills and treatment regimes to health care outcomes. But as yet little consideration is given in the medical journals to the substitution of non-medical for medical staff, or to the relative costs and benefits of varying the mix of health practitioners.

The concentration of national manpower planning on the aggregate supply and demand for physicians, as well as the particular interpretation given to medical demand, does enable precise forecasts to be made about the likely balance between supply and demand. What is rather less evident is whether the increased sophistication in manpower forecasting that has apparently been achieved will easily translate into policy interventions at the level of individual Health Authorities.

PRODUCTION OF PHYSICIANS

As in many health care systems, control of the recruitment, basic and continuing education of physicians is not exercised by the NHS or the DHSS alone. Instead there are a variety of formal and informal arrangements with other government departments, educational and professional groups.

For example, the Secretary of State for Education and Science has overall responsibility, through the University Grants Commission (UGC) for the provision and funding of medical school places. Joint funding is a well-established feature of medical education, as are the activities of several 'multi-interest' working groups such as the Education Liaison Group, and the Committee of Vice Chancellors and Principals.

Individual medical schools are responsible for undergraduate recruitment, and for the content and examination of medical education. However, the level of intake to individual schools is heavily influenced by the central Health Departments and the UGC, and even the undergraduate curriculum is subject to significant informal professional review and consultation. The medical profession has always regarded postgraduate medical education as even more directly controlled by its various colleges and professional bodies. The role of the central Health Departments is seen as financially facilitating professional goals, while also being keen to relate such postgraduate training to the Departments' own policies for the health services. At the postgraduate level, there is then a concerted effort to ensure regular contact between interested bodies - such as the General Medical Council (GMC), the Council for Postgraduate Medical Education (CPGME), Royal Colleges and Faculties, Universities, and more besides. The presence of the DHSS is also importantly felt through its responsibilities for allocating funds to the NHS Authorities.

Medical manpower production, in terms of both numbers and types of physician, therefore engages a variety of interests and in ways which are often regarded as crucial. The focus on the production dimension is most obvious in the continuing concern with the level of the medical school intake. The formulation and implementation of health manpower plans is often severely constrained by the lack of consensus across health manpower planners in central Health Departments and local Health Authorities and those in the educational and professional sectors. Each of these interested parties has on occasion the potential to frustrate or even veto central decisions not to their liking.

Closer examination of specific issues in medical education will illustrate these general points. There has been a continuing interest through the life of the NHS in the question: 'what sort of doctor are we trying to produce?' That

interest is evident, *inter alia*, in a Royal
Commission (Todd Report, 1968) and various
professional initiatives, such as the working
parties set up by the Royal College of General
Practitioners in 1980 and 1982 (RCGP, 1981; and
1985). The central aim of basic medical education
has been to train students to a common standard,
after which differing programmes of vocational and
postgraduate training prepare the doctor for
specialisation in a particular brand of medicine.
To enter general practice it is now necessary to
undertake three years of vocational training in the
NHS, and recent proposals from the RCGP Working
Party (1985) argue for further professional controls
to improve training and practice standards. Similar
adaptations in the undergraduate medical curricula
have proceeded apace over the years. The GMC (via
its education committee) has powers vested in it
through successive Medical Acts to regulate the
undergraduate curricula content, and has used this
authority, for example, to increase the amount of
social and behavioural sciences taught.

More central to the focus of this book is the
extent to which primary health care (PHC) has found
its way into British medical education. Medical
schools have widely been charged with inertia and
resistance to changing conditions in contemporary
society (Kaprio, 1979). It is significant, for
example, that the Royal College of General
Practitioner's own development of scenarios for
future primary care pays no direct attention to
'Health for All' (RCGP, 1985). A survey of primary
health care in medical education conducted in 1983
emphasised that Britain's lack of progress was
fairly typical across Europe (Walton, 1985). While
primary medical care was included in the
undergraduate curriculum it might not entail more
than relatively short work with, or lectures on,
general practice. It rarely extended to encompass
primary health care, and a focus on prevention
and the wider aspects of patient involvement in and
responsibility for their own health (pp.175-7).
Moreover, medical students and other trainee health
practitioners are not taught together in ways which
might facilitate subsequent inter-disciplinary
teamwork. Perhaps it is less surprising that
primary health care has such a low profile in
British medical education when the survey reports
that neither teachers nor the government show more
than lukewarm enthusiasm for sponsoring the aims
contained in the Alma-Ata Declaration.

'(H)alf of the most senior teachers of primary medical care, the heads of departments of general practice in the United Kingdom medical schools ... conveyed that they were unaware of the Alma-Ata Declaration, and of the place which primary health care is accorded as a concept in future improvement of health care services' (p.186).

While Walton suggests that medical ignorance of the Alma-Ata Declaration is the main reason for lack of progress towards establishing primary health care in the medical curriculum, there are also strong grounds for suspecting that it is not a development which commends itself to the medical community as a whole. However, some GPs appreciate that the emphasis on primary care offers important opportunities to advance their specialism and standing within the profession vis-a-vis their hospital colleagues.

This links with a further complaint made against basic medical education that it is overly 'mechanistic' and 'disease centred'. This is encouraged by its hospital orientation so that,

'students almost invariably see patients in bed, separated from home and family, under the care of specialists who are often mainly interested in the rare and complicated aspects of the problem' (WHO, 1985c, p.14).

Insofar as this approach does not facilitate the status of primary health care among medical students, it instead encourages a bias towards further medical specialisation. As specialities multiply, so the prescribed lengths of postgraduate training increase - with evident consequences for the production of physicians.

The expansion and sub-division of specialist training has raised considerable problems in order to ensure that physicians of the desired spread of specialisms are available at the time and in the quantities that local Health Authorities require. Again, this is an area where close collaboration between educational institutions, professional bodies, central Health Departments and local Health Authorities is crucial. Yet the continuing experience has been that medical students gravitate towards more popular specialisms - such as surgery and internal medicine - and leave in their wake a group of 'shortage specialties' - such as geriatrics and mental illness. In the main what progress there has been towards improving the match of specialty demand and supply has been achieved by central limits on approval of consultant and training posts. A significant number of unfilled posts remain but no other effective scheme has been found to induce junior doctors to opt for the less favoured specialties (House of Commons, 1985a). The direction of physicians into shortage specialisms or areas has not commended itself to the profession.

'The DHSS's view is that career guidance and information on career prospects, together with a selective creation of additional training posts, are the best ways of filling shortages and meeting priorities' (NAO, 1985a, p.10).

It is a feature of health manpower production in the NHS that there are several major 'players' who each have significant and not always compatible interests to promote. Effective collaboration is not for the want of regular joint discussions and working parties to explore medical education and training. Yet the problems of medical manpower production extend beyond the difficulties of co-ordinating the various interest groups. Given the lack and future uncertainty of resources, and the multiplication of service priorities, the integration of appropriate educational policies with service development remains an elusive goal.

MEDICAL MANPOWER MANAGEMENT

The central focus of health manpower management needs to lie in a capacity to bring health care practitioner and organisational goals into close harmony (Mejia, 1978, p.39). This pinpoints a major area of dispute between central Health Departments and local Health Authorities, and the medical profession. It is moreover a subject which has gained increased prominence in health policy deliberations. Earlier discussion has already highlighted the growing pressure on Health Authorities and the medical profession to take more heed of budgetary constraints, and additionally to examine existing practices and future plans, in the light of priorities and needs, in order to determine the most efficient and effective health services. Over the life of the NHS, the prime context in which the management of medical manpower has been considered has been the career structure. This continues to be at the heart of most professional discussion. Some aspects of these debates are explored in this section to indicate how 'management' problems can be so divisive in the NHS.

There has been a succession of reports and inquiries into medical and dental hospital staffing which pre-date the inception of the NHS. These have been dominated by representatives from central Health Departments, local Health Authorities and the various professional bodies. Through the period since the 1940s, the medical profession has concentrated its attention on the hospital career structure, education and training. The recommendations of the Spens Report of 1948 formed the basis for hospital staffing arrangements. After registration with the General Medical Council, medical graduates had to pass through several training grades before achieving the position of hospital consultant. In practice, imbalances across the grades have been a continuing source of professional concern. The Platt Report of 1961 emphasised the problems inherent in a system which sought to satisfy both the service needs of the NHS and the training and career aspirations of physicians. Some of its suggestions for selective changes in the training grades were subsequently implemented, including a new sub-consultant grade of Medical Assistant (since re-named Associate Specialist), and a Hospital Practitioner grade for those training to become General Practitioners.

The Platt Report also suggested a more fundamental change in the career structure of hospital staff which would have established a new permanent sub-consultant career grade. The Royal Commission on Medical Education (Todd Report, 1968) added its own support for such a grade with a measure of clinical autonomy. Variations of this theme continue to be aired within the medical profession. For example, the Royal Commission on the National Health Service (Report, 1979) re-iterated the 'need for improvement in the hospital career structure for doctors' (para.14.84) but abstained from making 'a recommendation in this difficult and contentious area' (para.14.92). Instead it outlined 'a possible alternative' in an Appendix. This suggested a simplified staffing structure - assistant physician, physician and consultant physician. Below the consultant grade as

presently understood would be a physician grade,
itself sub-divided into 'training' and 'career'
positions. This latter category would essentially
comprise sub-consultants with specific clinical
responsibilities, and some of these would be
promoted to consultant physician grade.
Nevertheless, the profession as a whole has firmly
resisted any such innovation. The internal
divisions and entrenched position of the Royal
Colleges make it difficult to identify or organise a
common 'medical' interest for change.

More general agreement was reached between the
central Health Departments and the professions that
immediate action had to be taken to correct the
worsening imbalances in the hospital staffing
structure. In three 'Progress Reports' from the
late 1960s and early 1970s the preferred policy
options entailed: a general expansion in hospital
staff of 3% per year, although faster for
consultants (4%) than for juniors (2.5%); the length
of time in postgraduate training should be based on
educational criteria alone; and attempts should
generally be directed towards ensuring greater
equilibrium between medical and dental school
output, those in training grades, and consultant
openings (DHSS, 1985a). Despite this agreement and
the controls on junior doctor posts imposed by the
Central Manpower Committee the expansion of juniors
between 1971 and 1980 was 50%, and the growth of
consultants only 28% (NAO, 1985a, para.4.8). While
the medical profession sought unsuccessfully to
generate its own proposals (Brearley, 1984), the
House of Commons Social Services Select Committee
began its own investigation in 1980 into 'Medical
Education - with special reference to the number of
doctors and the career structure in hospitals'
(1981). This Short Report gave full backing for
moves towards a 'consultant-provided' rather than a
'consultant-led' service. It recommended a
significant increase in the number of consultants
and a reduction in the number of junior doctors.
The government welcomed this strategy and the DHSS
(HC(82)4) set down three separate but related
targets to facilitate this changed balance in the
hospital staffing structure:

1   double the number of consultants in the next
    15 years;
2   reverse the current ratio of 1.8 juniors to
    every consultant by the year 2,000; and
3   achieve parity between junior doctors and

consultants by 1988.

The general intention was both to improve the level of care provided to patients, and to enhance the career prospects of medical graduates. There was a further suggestion that a consultant-provided service would also secure a more efficient and effective use of resources.

While some sections of the profession welcomed the government's intervention as generally appropriate, there was also a noticeably lukewarm, and at times downright hostile, reaction from important sections of the medical establishment - consultants, BMA, and Royal Colleges. For many the projected change in consultants' working conditions looked excessive and demeaning: 'such a change implies ... "shift" medicine, flexible rostering, and residence in hospital for the rest of many consultants' working lives' (Appleyard, 1982, p.1355). Others forecast the end of the consultant as the head of a junior doctor 'firm'. Nevertheless, the government was adamant. In HC(82)4 Health Authorities were asked to freeze expansion of Senior House Officer posts in England and Wales - as had already been done in Scotland. Furthermore, RHAs were requested to draw up plans for achieving the intended target of consultant-junior doctor parity by 1988. As an additional stimulus to action, this was included as a topic for consideration in the new system of Annual Planning Reviews.

Since 1981 the whole-time-equivalent (WTE) ratio of consultants to juniors has fallen marginally from 1:1.77 to 1:1.69 in 1984, but there is little prospect of reaching parity by 1988. The National Audit Office report on hospital based medical manpower concluded:

> '(t)here appears to be a conflict between Departmental policy to increase the proportion of consultant posts - broadly agreed with the profession centrally, and implementation by Health Authorities subject to pressure from local professional interests' (NAO, 1985a, para.4.21).

In its own follow-up report, the Social Services Select Committee found that Regional plans for achieving the consultant-provided service gave little grounds for optimism (House of Commons, 1985a). A combination of medical opposition to a marked reduction in junior doctor numbers, a change in the character of consultants' work, and a shortage of cash to effect a significant increase in the number of consultants have been emphasised as the main reasons for the lack of progress. The Health Minister downgraded the targets 'as signposts pointing in the right direction' (ibid, p.viii), and not likely to be achieved in the NHS by the 1990s. The government's enthusiasm which in large part was stimulated by claims about significant cost savings, has been tempered by the absence of detailed research confirming the efficiency and effectiveness of a change in the grade mix of hospital medical staff.

As an exercise in manpower planning and management, the consultant-junior ratio debate aptly illustrates the gap that exists between theory and practice. For all the increasingly sophisticated forecasting exercises in which central Health Departments have engaged, they have not spelt out how the targetted ratio has to be determined - whether between consultants and juniors, or across specialisms.

In similar fashion, the professional response to suggestions in the Short Report (1981) that there should be a wider experimentation with doctor-substitution and multi-disciplinary teams has found little favour. Although the National Audit Office Report (1985a) accepted local Health Authorities' claims that, 'experimentation continues in the use of non-medical grades for work normally carried out by doctors, and of multi-disciplinary teams' (para.3.17), no concrete examples were offered, nor was any indication given of the extent of schemes designed to increase the efficient utilisation of staff. There has been growing interest in deriving workload and performance measures but these have little application at the local level in planning across medical specialties, and none at all in comparing different staff groups.

It is also noticeable that there have been few initiatives to exploit any flexibility in the remuneration and conditions of service of physicians in order to serve wider manpower and health service goals. A fixed number of distinction and meritorious service awards are provided for NHS consultants, and in 1983 there were just over 6,000 recipients - or 35.7% of those eligible (para. 5.5). However, there is nothing in the criteria which would improve the financial prospects of those in the shortage specialisms - indeed the awards have gone in large part to those which are most oversupplied with prospective consultants. Another illustration is that consultants contracts are with RHAs, and GPs' contracts with Family Practitioners Committees (FPCs). This leaves little scope for managerial intervention by local Health Authorities. Recommendations for changes in the remuneration structure, and in contractual terms and conditions of service, are securely in the hands of the profession and the Health Departments. Neither has made serious overtures to drastically change the present system, despite the widespread calls to make the management of medical services more efficient.

The Royal College of General Practitioners has however taken some steps towards supporting schemes which reward those GPs who provide a better quality service than their peers (RCGP, 1985). Their concern is both directed towards improving the performance of GPs as well as opening up the possibility of distinction awards for those providing 'better' primary care. The reaction from the British Medical Association has been generally hostile. The central Health Departments have not reacted with any marked enthusiasm - preferring instead to increase the accountability of GPs by encouraging the FPCs to take a more interventionist role. Examples of this line of approach are to be seen in the use by some FPCs of GP facilitators and programmes to inspect GP premises. These initiatives aside it is noticeable that there are no long term strategic plans for primary health care services as are required for most hospital services; this may change with the recent publication of a discussion paper on manpower and service delivery patterns in PHC (DHSS, 1986b). At present FPCs can make policy statements but they can seldom enforce their priorities - in large part because GPs enjoy an even more 'independent' status than their hospital colleagues.

The discussion of medical manpower management therefore returns to the distinctive 'unmanaged status' of so much medical activity in the NHS. That ensures a continuing contradiction between the professional aspirations to enhance the medical career structure, and attempts to manage the health services in ways which accord primacy to some other organisational goals.

INTEGRATING THE MANPOWER PROCESS

The all too frequent lack of co-ordination among the
several interests concerned with the planning,
production and management of medical manpower has
been a recurring theme in this discussion. It
constitutes a major problem in improving the quality
of the manpower process from the formulation of
plans to their implementation and evaluation. The
root cause has been presented as a conflict between
professional autonomy and public accountability. It
is further in evidence in the problematic relationship between the central and local levels of the
health service. This latter dimension has gained
increased prominence as the central authorities have
taken repeated initiatives to improve the state of
health manpower planning in general, and medical
manpower planning in particular. How far, and in
what ways, this stimulus from the centre has brought
an end to the widely recognised isolation of medical
manpower from wider service planning is much
debated.

The largely token presence of local medical
manpower planning is still widely acknowledged - not
least by Regional Medical Officers. For example,
Todd (1983; 1985) has explored in some detail how,
in her experience as a district general manager,
medical manpower planning is widely viewed as a 'no-
go' area. It is a considerable achievement to get
those in the health service to jointly discuss such
questions as:

- what sort of work should different grades
  of medical staff be able to undertake?
- what grade mix is most appropriate?
- how far does this vary across specialties?
- what is the relationship between costs
  and outcomes in medical care?

The general impression is that professional
resistance to further management of their sphere of
interest has not been overcome to any significant
degree as advocated by central decision makers. NAO
(1985a) concluded that 'medical manpower planning
at both regional and district level was not very
advanced' (para.2.10). Further, 'in the absence of
co-ordinated planning, most DHAs were forced to try
to meet the health needs of the local community as
and when they arose' (para.2.10) - rather than
through a careful integration of medical manpower

planning with projected service developments. The
problem is that while national forecasts are made
about total numbers of medical staff, it is left to
the local level to 'translate this into medical
manpower requirements by specialty and to ensure
that there will be an adequate supply of doctors
with the right skills to meet these requirements'
(para.2.14).

There exists very little proven wisdom on which
to base such an exercise. Some instructive
descriptions of local medical manpower planning have
nevertheless recently appeared in the health
services literature (Parkhouse and O'Brien, 1984;
Todd, 1985; Coyne, 1985; Allen, 1986). The
assumption on which the Northern Region attempted to
establish consultant needs by local evaluation has
been widely commended (Parkhouse and O'Brien, 1984).
Yet no easy solution has been found to balance the
often different interpretation of medical needs at
local and higher tiers. The charge is frequently
levelled that national agreements are not introduced
in the Districts because the necessary information,
encouragement and resources are lacking. Instances
are cited where a Region received an allocation of
consultants in quite different specialties to those
earmarked in local service developments (Carruthers,
1984). There is obvious competition within and
between Regions, as well as between the central
authorities and local bodies; this has not been
eliminated by the introduction of a holistic
planning system. To some degree, this has served to
institutionalise and aggravate professional-
managerial rivalries within and between levels.

It is in the pages of the professional journals
that the lack of enthusiasm for a fully integrated
health manpower process is clearly revealed.
The manpower process as an activity does not commend
itself to the profession, except insofar as
imbalances in the demand and supply of physicians
create confusion and disorder in the medical career
structure. The profession approaches the subject
from a position of some strength: because of its
significance in the delivery and organisation of
health care; its jealously guarded occupational
control; and its public role as defender of the
public-patient interest. It is therefore able to
exert an important veto power in thwarting health
policies which it dislikes. The position is further
complicated because even professional organisations
find difficulties at times in binding their members
to agreements made with central Health Departments.

Such is the independence of individual physicians, and the significant rivalries within the medical community. All of these dimensions come through strongly in an examination of medical manpower. Acceptance of the WHO strategy for 'planning, producing and managing health personnel to work as teams in well planned services adapted to local conditions' (Fulop, 1982, p.4) still seems a distant goal on the NHS horizon.

Chapter 5

NURSES AND NURSING

As the largest single group of NHS employees, nurses
expect to figure prominently in manpower reviews.
It is the size and differentiation of the nursing
workforce, along with the volume of its budget,
which provide the initial contexts for understanding
the attempts to control nurse manpower in the NHS.
Not surprisingly, the profession has been mindful of
the threats and opportunities posed by the general
growth of managerialism in the health services.
Close scrutiny by 'outsiders' is frequently resented
by a group which wishes to advance its professional
status and occupational control. The commitment of
nurses to management structures in general and to
manpower processes in particular reflects the
profession's view that through greater self
management – using opportunities recently provided –
they will be better able to advance and defend the
nursing interest. The nursing contribution to the
manpower process is therefore alternately excited
and threatened by the prospects it offers.
     In the following discussion particular
attention is devoted to the ways in which the
profession has confronted the technical demands to
'think manpower'. But it is also crucial to
appreciate the political context in which nursing
engages with manpower issues: as a prism through
which it perceives its professional standing
relative to other health care practitioners in the
NHS. Most revealingly, a comparison of the main
objectives set down for the recent National Audit
Office Reports (1985a; 1985b) on physicians and
nurses reveals the extent to which medical dominance
in the NHS can orient manpower investigations to a
professional concern with the hospital career
structure, while comparable debates in nursing are
almost entirely ignored. The larger degree of
control exercised by the central Health Departments
and local Health Authorities is conveyed by the

inclusion in the nursing report alone of the objective to consider:

'whether or not the evidence suggested that the NHS deployed the right numbers and grades of nursing staff in the most efficient and effective manner' (1985b, p.1).

No equivalent focus on the management and utilisation of medical staff was pursued.

In consequence, discussion of manpower initiatives takes a different form, and reaches a higher level of 'technical' sophistication in nursing compared with medicine. It has also given fresh momentum and urgency to what has been a long-running self-evaluation within the profession about the role of nurses in the care of patients, and in the general management of the health services.

PLANNING: NURSING STOCKS AND FLOWS

There have been a series of inquiries into aspects of the planning, production and management of nursing and nurses. The Report of the Committee on Nursing (Briggs Report, 1972) offered a comprehensive review of past discussions and current thinking on the role of the nurse and how nursing might be better managed. This highlighted shortcomings in nurse manpower planning, as did the Royal Commission on the National Health Service (Report, 1979), although nursing did not compare unfavourably with other staff groups. As the nursing profession embraced the new management and planning structures, manpower planning acquired its own designated nurse managers. Furthermore, the central Health Departments have been instrumental in fostering the notion of nurse manpower planning, enhancing its technical sophistication and information base (DHSS, 1982a; 1983d).

Few groups have so obviously found themselves in the midst of recurring mismatches in the supply of and demand for staff as nurses. Periods of staff surplus have interchanged with periods of shortage. Throughout these years the task of ensuring that the right number of nurses with the required skills were available at the local level has been the cause of constant frustration. Unlike for physicians, the DHSS has not organised national forecasts for nurse supply and demand. It has instead relied on local Health Authorities to devise their own projections on the basis of service plans. Since 1979, the DHSS has been able to monitor nurse numbers through the strategic planning exercise, along with the quarterly returns on staff in post provided by RHAs since 1983. The Health Departments have also taken policy decisions which indicate that central control has not lapsed. Cash limits have been imposed as well as manpower cuts. Furthermore, recent initiatives to strengthen general management are likely to weaken the role of nurse managers (Rowden, 1985; Buchan, 1985; Rogers, 1986).

An indication that local manpower planning was expected to put its own house in order was demonstrated by the establishment of the Manpower Planning Advisory Group (MPAG) in 1983 which included in its programme the development of demand methodologies for use by nurse managers, as well as a national supply model. The NAO Report (1985b, part 3) implied that there were too many nurses; it pointed to the lack of any systematic determination of the 16% increase in nursing and midwifery between 1976 and 1983. However, a substantial part of the additional staff had been recruited as a direct result of the increase in holiday allowances and especially with the reduction of the working week from forty to thirty seven and a half hours. Furthermore, according to the DHSS's own calculations, there has been an increased demand for nursing services over this period, with more intensive use of acute service beds as well as a growth in admissions of those highly dependent on nursing care, such as the elderly. The dynamics of service needs have also led to a shift in the balance of care from the hospital to the community with important consequences for the organisation of nursing resources.

Demand

The question 'how many nurses are needed?' has given rise to numerous methodologies which carry the exercise through to often very precise detail. These have been sponsored by the central Health Departments, within local Health Authorities, and on the initiative of local groups of nurse managers. The traditional method of using 'norms' for establishment levels has come under general attack for its reliance on historical staffing levels which 'had rarely been adapted to take account of changes in service plans, working practices or changes in demographic patterns' (NAO, 1985b, para.3.3). The

DHSS has not felt able to endorse any alternative method as the one 'best' solution for estimating nursing requirements, but has instead approved a number of options, which alone, or in combination, should aid nurse planners (DHSS, 1984a).

The methods for determining nursing staff needs are generally categorised as 'top down' or 'bottom up'. 'Top down' methods relate patient needs and nursing personnel through a variety of measures - but especially through the use of norms of staff per bed, per head of population, or per type of patient. An example is the British Geriatric Society's target of one nurse per 1.25 geriatric in-patients. Other widely referenced schemes include the Trent method, the Revenue Consequences of Capital Schemes (RCCS) formula, Rhys Hearn and Auld's method. The Aberdeen formula provides another example, at least in the way it operates in practice, as opposed to the way it was researched. These are based on: regression analysis; statistical averages; and activity sampling related to patient dependency. 'Bottom up' methods are generated locally on the basis of professional judgement of what is required. GRASP, Criteria For Care and MONITOR, and the Telford, Cheltenham and Goddard methods have all received wide discussion in the manpower planning literature. They are based on measures of activity analysis, dependency and professional judgement (see Table 5.1).

The majority of recent schemes is based on a 'bottom up' methodology. This highlights the importance of professional judgement at the clinical and local managerial level. As Bloore (1984) commented with respect to the Cheltenham method, it was devised to provide analytical support for subjective views and professional judgement. Such approaches are very much in tune with contemporary criticism of the 'top down' methods on the grounds that there is little attempt to incorporate workload measures, poor flexibility (to allow, for example, for contrasting local policies on admissions and discharges) and a lack of consultation with the nursing staff. The DHSS's (1984a) own investigation of 'top down' and 'bottom up' procedures acknowledged the difficulties in evaluating the merits of the different approaches - both between and within the two main camps.

The NAO investigation of 16 District Health Authorities found that:

Table 5.1: Nurse Demand Methodologies

	Approach Top Down	Approach Bottom Up	Specialty	Main Method(s) of Measurement	Based on Individual Care	Standard of Care Monitored	Based on Professional Judgement	Identifies Staff Mix
RCCS Formula	Yes	-	All	Statistical averages	Low	Low	Low	Low
British Geriatric Society Norm	Yes	-	Geriatrics	Statistical	Low	Low	Low	Low
Aberdeen	Yes	-	Acute, Mid-wifery, Geriatrics	Activity sampling related to dependency	Low	Low	Low	Low
Auld	Yes	-	Midwifery	Activity analysis and self-recording	Low	Low	Medium	Low
Trent	Yes	-	All	Statistical regression analysis	Low	Low	Low	Low
Rhys Hearn	Yes	-	Geriatrics	Workload related to dependency	High	Medium	Medium	Medium
Cheltenham	-	Yes	General	Activity analysis, consensus of opinion and dependency	Medium	Low	High	Medium
GRASP	-	Yes	Acute, Psychiatry Geriatrics	Activity analysis and consensus of opinion	High	High	High	Medium
Criteria for Care and MONITOR	-	Yes	Medical and Surgical	Activity analysis dependency, and measurement of quality	Low	High	Medium	Low
Telford	-	Yes	All	Not quantitative	Low	Low	High	Medium

Sources: Illsley and Goldstone, 1985, p.15; All Wales Committee, 1985, p.12.

'In three Health Authorities no attempt had been made by nurse managers to assess by use of some recognised methodology the number of nursing staff required ... while at the remaining thirteen Authorities the managers used a variety of 'bottom up' and 'top down' methods. In six Authorities ... the number of staff in post was lower than both the nursing manpower requirement determined by the use of the various methodologies and also "funded establishment", which is usually interpreted by the NHS as the number of nurses the district could afford ....' (1985b, para.3.14).

It also highlighted the capacity of the 'top down' mode to arrive at a demand for nursing staff below the number currently employed in the authorities' reviewed (p.12). In terms of professional acceptability, 'top down' methods enjoyed little favour. But the DHSS maintained that these have their uses in certain situations; their response was couched in terms that nursing establishments were not ungenerous, and that the various methodologies also erred on the generous side in determining nursing manpower (para.3.15).

The greater enthusiasm in the nursing profession for 'bottom up' techniques spans several issues. They are perceived as a means to provide greater professional involvement and control over the nursing establishment. Further, by questioning historical staffing arrangements the methods are seen to be more in tune with changing nursing practices. 'Top down' approaches have been biased towards a task-oriented nursing regime which has been retreating before the 'nursing process' view of patient care (Illsley and Goldstone, 1985, p.16). Not least, nurse managers have been searching for a method which was both acceptable in professional terms and which generated sophisticated data for planning at district, unit and ward levels. There is a widespread perception among nurses that they are, as a group, under particular pressure to put staffing forecasts on a more defensible footing. '... It is necessary for nurses at all levels to justify their needs by validated analysis' (Bloore, 1984, p.57). There has been a growing confidence in these methodologies because they have provided a credible basis for defending existing staffing levels, and in some cases have been used to justify increased nursing establishments.

The 'bottom up' methodologies have though not

gone uncriticised among nurses. The time and resources required to institute these methods varies greatly. For example, both GRASP and the Cheltenham method require extended examination of workload levels, activity analysis and professional opinion. The aim is to ensure nurse involvement and commitment, but the complexities in patient care are such that there will always be scope for disagreement. For example, physical aspects of care are more easily measured than the psycho-social. Nevertheless the planning constraint is to support professional judgement with 'objective' data. Similar issues surround the inclusion of quality control: whether of nurse or patient satisfaction. For instance, the Criteria for Care and MONITOR method includes both workload and service quality measures. The latter entails division of patients into four dependency groups - ranging from maximum to minimum care. Single 'yes/no' questions are then posed against four aspects of the nursing care: planning and assessment; physical care; non-physical care; and evaluation of care. Given the pressures also building up to increase quality assurance among health professionals, this approach has found increasing support (All Wales Nurse Manpower Planning Committee, 1985, para.2.10).

The majority of these demand techniques have been designed for the hospital setting, and sometimes specific nursing areas within the acute sector. In contrast, the estimation of demand for community nurses has remained in a traditional mould - on a nurse-per-population ratio basis. There is a general consensus that community nursing requires its own approach. While hospital workload is largely generated by consultants, in the community GPs are but one of several factors which impact on manpower allocations, costs and service objectives. It is also the case that nursing services in the community cover a particularly wide range of skills, and not all would accept the general 'nurse' designation: district nurses, health visitors, midwives, community nursing for the mentally ill and handicapped, school and other specialist nurses (NAO, 1985b, p.13). The DHSS has issued what it termed 'yardsticks' of adequate community care, although these were distinguished from 'standards' or 'norms', because of the need to adapt to specific local conditions. For example, a health visitor ratio that ranged from 1:4,300 to 1:3,000 was endorsed, while the ratio for district nurses spread between 1:2,500 to 1:4,000. In September 1983, 65%

of Health Authorities had failed to reach the
yardsticks of 1:4,600 for health visitors which had
been set down in 1972 although only 8% had not
attained the district nursing figure of 1:4,000.
Furthermore, none of those Authorities which were by
these indicators 'underprovided' had attempted to
evaluate how far, and in what ways, health status in
the community had suffered as a consequence
(para.3.19). The London Health Planning
Consortium's (LHPC) Report (1981) suggested that
primary care standards were indeed falling, but
despite further inquiries no fresh yardsticks for
community nursing have been introduced.

This theme is taken up in the Cumberlege Report
on Neighbourhood Nursing (DHSS, 1986a). A switch in
resources from the hospital services is advocated
although it recognises that the manpower and cost
implications of this policy are either not available
or 'confusing' (pp.52-3). The report refrains from
specifying national norms and instead lays
particular emphasis on ensuring that 'the health
needs of individuals and communities are properly
identified' (p.2).

> 'If primary care is to be relevant and achieve
> the goals set by the World Health Organization
> for the Year 2000 there must be a greater move
> to considering the whole person's well being
> and in this the community nurse excels'
> (Foreword).

To this end, neighbourhood teams are expected to
build up their own 'population profile'.

This implies a modification of population-to-
nurse ratios with information which:

> '... should show demography trends, the
> patterns and trends in morbidity and the
> neighbourhood's social and environmental
> characteristics' (p.18).

The bottom up approaches which have won such favour
among hospital based nurse managers, especially in
so far as they allow an input for professional
judgement, have few parallels in the community
services. For example, activity analysis and
measures of workload related to dependency have
proven most difficult to formulate - not least
because of the more general caring, preventive and
health promotion role of the community services.
The report acknowledges that estimating the demand

for community services is additionally complicated by the fragmentation of professional roles - for example, between health visitors, district nurses and school nurses. While the role of specialist nurses in the community is supported, a radical organisation of training and education is also called for to provide a more flexible workforce and thereby to lessen some of the existing difficulties in providing a balance between supply and demand for community staff.

Forecasts of the demand for nursing staff, whether based on 'top down' or 'bottom up' approaches, have been difficult to operate in Authorities hard pressed for financial resources. Such planning has been further hindered because of the difficulties in relating different staffing levels or mixes of nursing staff with patient care and cost outcomes. Hence forecasts of demand for particular types of nurse, or of qualified and unqualified staff, are conspicuous by their absence from the nurse manpower literature.

It is interesting to note that the DHSS has not set national guidelines on the mix of nursing staff, whereas in Scotland, the Aberdeen formula has been recommended for use by the Scottish Home and Health Department (SHHD). The English National Board has however suggested that greater attention should be given to the ratio of qualified staff to learners, in large part because the latter has been crucial to the delivery of direct nursing care although comprising a minority of the nursing workforce. The balance of service and training needs has traditionally been heavily stacked in favour of the cheap labour which learners provide.

Instances where unqualified staff and/or learners have been alone on wards, especially in psychiatric and geriatric units, have been frequently reported. The Royal Commission on the National Health Service (Report, 1979) commented on the lack of research evidence about the most appropriate composition of the nursing staff that served both service and education needs. Over the last decade the grade composition of the nursing establishment has altered, with a 4% reduction in learners, compared with a 14% growth in unqualified staff, and a 27% increase in qualified nurses. This meant a 56:20:24 ratio of qualified nurses to learners to unqualified personnel. The NAO Report (1985b) stated that the general nursing aim was to increase the qualified complement to 60%, although as with the ratio of consultants to junior doctors there seemed to be no sophisticated manpower calculations underlying this target.

The demand for nurses has not been reinterpreted, at least directly, to the extent of available resources as with physicians. However, that link cannot be ignored. The response varies across Authorities. Nursing establishments may be kept low, and the grade mix may be balanced towards learners and unqualified staff. The demand for nursing staff is therefore more amenable to local definition and reinterpretation than is the case with physicians. At the same time, there appears to be no discussion focussing on the need for an aggregate increase in nurses. While there is mention of the impact of demographic factors, changing nursing practices, and improvements in the quality of services provided, the general impression conveyed by central Health Departments is that no overall increase in nursing manpower is required.

Supply

In contrast to the consideration given to estimating the demand for nurses relatively little attention or enthusiasm is currently generated by supply side issues. In large part this is related to the current economic situation which has encouraged lower rates of nurse turnover as well as policies within some Authorities to restrict nurse establishments.

The DHSS has taken an interest in developing a supply model, but most initiatives have been conducted at the local level by nurse managers and manpower planners. This contrast with medicine reflects the fact that responsibility for recruitment to nursing schools and to nursing posts in the NHS lies with local Health Authorities. For the most part there is a wide gulf between national and local information. Some progress has been made towards establishing a UKCC register of qualified staff which provides a picture of total numbers as well as the distribution across specialties, but this is a professional register only, with no right of access to those outside the UKCC. In addition, there are always problems in knowing what proportion of this pool of staff is currently in post or available for employment. There are further difficulties in breaking down these national supply figures to even the Regional level. While information is available on learner intake levels (these stood at 26,000 in England and Wales in 1984, having fallen from 37,000 in 1979) and on wastage rates (these have fallen to under 10% over the same period), the calculations on which the pool of nurses is being increased seem little more than the sum of local decisions. This begs the question of how far the supply net for nurses stretches – geographically, between the NHS and other potential employers, and across different parts of the health service. Supply issues in community nursing offer a similar picture. At the present time, most Authorities do not appear to be experiencing special problems (DHSS 1986a, p.52). However, there are some Regional disparities which tend to replicate those in the hospital services. Recruitment also varies between professional staff groups. For example, health visiting is over-supplied with potential applicants, while district nursing reports some recruitment difficulties (p.52). The Cumberlege Report concluded that the most significant supply question for community nursing was that well-qualified applicants were being rejected because of a shortage of training places or a lack of sponsorship from Health Authorities (p.52).

The recruitment into nurse training has become somewhat more specialised in recent years with a concentration on those with General Certificate of Education Ordinary and Advanced levels. As approximately 90% of nurses are female, nursing recruitment is dependent on both demographic trends and the availability of alternative employment for young females (Long and Mercer, 1978). By the same token, the employment of nursing staff connects closely with labour market conditions. A particular issue is the opportunity for employment on a part-time basis, and this has also been a topic with regard to training courses. The paradox has often been noted that although nursing is a predominantly female profession it offers few opportunities for basic or post-basic training on a part-time basis – unlike medicine. Hutt (1984) has further suggested that part-time nurses have been regarded as second-best by nurse managers, despite lower turnover rates; a full-time workforce is considered the professional norm. In like fashion, the supply of working mothers has not been facilitated by the relative shortage of NHS creche and nursery places.

The general impression is that nurse managers do not feel it necessary, or do not feel that the results repay the effort, to closely monitor and exploit the local labour market for nursing staff. There are exceptions. Some Authorities have, for example, developed nurse banks in order to provide a flexible reserve in times of particular difficulty in nurse supply. It is initiatives such as nurse banks and staff creches however which fall first victim to expenditure cuts (Farrow, 1982).

The impact of debates through the 1970s about the level and character of nursing turnover had generally subsided only to be revived at the present time. The retention of experienced, qualified staff is far less of a problem in the mid 1980s compared with a decade ago. It is also apparent that the considerable mismatches in supply and demand have led to several initiatives to model the flow of nurses through a local system. These have been used to try and plan more carefully for the level of new recruitment, of both learners and already qualified staff, as well as their promotion, and levels of departure in order to minimise the fluctuations in supply. While discussions of supply side problems have pointed to several areas which require close attention, or where remedial action should be concentrated - turnover, sickness and absence levels, part-time working, flexible hours, nurse banks and re-training courses - the literature also highlights the important effect of factors outside the control of nurse managers - levels of economic activity, changing roles of women, and general labour market relativities.

Overall, both demand and supply side debates in nursing have generated even shares of optimism and pessimism. It is apparent across both contexts that the problems are extremely complex and the policy solutions far from certain in their effect. Once again the importance of professional acceptability of the methods is central to their success. But along with the need for professional approval there is abundant evidence that the nursing profession does not talk with one voice, so that as the demand methodologies illustrate, the variety of nursing skills inhibits the formulation of forecasts for the nursing profession as a whole.

PRODUCTION: EDUCATION AND TRAINING

Over the last few years numerous articles have appeared in the nursing press around the general theme that nursing is 'at the crossroads' (Boylan, 1982). Nowhere is this turmoil of professional concern more in evidence than in education and training priorities and policies. There has been both a continuing debate in the nursing press and a succession of professional and Health Department sponsored inquiries and reports about the ways in which the production of nurses should be conducted, and how this might be better co-ordinated with both the planning and management of nursing staff in the NHS. The trail runs from the <u>Hodder Report</u> (1943), through the <u>Wood Report</u> (1947), the <u>Platt Report</u> (1959), the <u>Briggs Report</u> (1972), discussion in the Royal Commission on the National Health Service <u>Report</u> (1979), up to the most recent contributions – the <u>Judge Report</u> from the RCN (1985), the English National Board's consultative document (ENB, 1985a) and the UKCC (1985a,b,c,d; 1986) initiative entitled <u>Project 2000</u>. The latter's initial recommendations are proclaimed as 'nothing less than a revolution in the usage of manpower in the NHS' (UKCC, 1986, p.66). It is most obviously also part of a long line of soul searching exercises within nursing about its professional standing and ambition – well summarised by one commentator in the phrase, 'from handmaiden to health specialist' (Draper, 1981). The emphasis has been on the special and distinctive skills and contribution that nurses bring to patient care. This is amply illustrated in the advocacy of the nursing process as comprising quite a specific theoretical and practical knowledge and approach that distinguishes nursing from other health professions (not least physicians), as well as drawing an emphatic dividing line between qualified nurse professionals and 'nursing' auxiliaries and aides – who so many in the profession consider should not carry the 'nurse' label.

The context in which the RCN, ENB and UKCC documents are set is one of the over-riding need to develop a strategy for nursing that will enable the profession to cope with changing health care demands:

> 'If the health demands of the population are to be properly met and the health services are not to be overwhelmed by the growing need for care, then nursing must not react to disease, but must be much more involved in helping people to achieve health more effectively' (ENB, 1985a, quoted in Bendall, 1985, p.53).

The emphasis is on a heightened role for nursing as there is a shift in health care from hospitals to the community. As originally formulated by the UKCC the five major questions for discussion in <u>Project 2000</u> were:

1 Is there a case for a generic nurse?
2 Should students be part of the workforce?
3 Where should training take place?
4 Should there be one level of nurse?
5 What reforms are needed for continuing education?
(Dickson, 1985, p.27)

There is a widespread feeling within nursing that it is imperative to expand the educational base of nursing and to introduce greater professional accountability at the individual level. The embrace of a more 'professional' approach in regard to education and training is regarded as crucial:

'... professions in our society exert powerful influences on moral and social changes - power and influence make up the strength of any organisation' (Dawe, 1984, p.28).

There is also abundant evidence from the nursing press that there are significant tensions and divisions within nursing. The increased concern with organising at the level of nurse specialism is indicative of the difficulty in generating a common stance on nurse education and training. Thus, while there is considerable enthusiasm for change, some groups face an uncertain future, which has exacerbated fissures within the profession.

A particular illustration of a group which considers itself under threat is midwifery. The Royal College of Midwives has been noticeably distancing itself from nursing in recent years, not just in terms of education and training, but in pay and management as well. For example, midwives and registered sick children's nurses (RSCNs) have been in dispute about their respective competences and responsibilities for neo-natal care (Newson, 1982). Midwives have also campaigned vigorously against what they see as the medical profession's take-over and (mis)understanding of the birthing process.

'The midwife has been maligned and discredited as a professional, the erosion and contraction of her function and under-utilisation of her skills are well documented facts' (Towler, 1982, p.2).

There have been charges that they are in danger of being transformed into family planning advisers.

The midwives' complaints also contain a defence of a woman's right to choose and control the birth process, and a rejection of male, medical and overly technological hospital interests. A return to home confinements and a greater patient involvement in the management of pregnancy and birthing are regarded as running parallel to the midwives' background and training. So it is argued that midwives must be prepared to act as autonomous professionals in clinical areas. Midwives have increasingly supported moves to give expectant mothers more continuity and control of their pregnancy through midwifery, rather than consultant units, as well as calling for an expansion of the community midwifery service to support home confinements (Towler, 1982; Willmott, 1980; DHSS, 1986a). A developing theme in the <u>Midwifery, Health Visitor and Community Nurse</u> journal has been that midwives should be educated to become independent practitioners within the NHS, with their own caseload. This highlights inter- and intra-professional rivalries in the health field. It also leads to suggestions for direct entry into midwifery courses, and brings midwives' ambitions into direct conflict with those advocating a common foundation across nursing and midwifery.

The experience of midwives is not exceptional. Comparable debates have surrounded the education and training of other groups. The case for a generic nurse - a 'nurse of all trades' (Kratz, 1985) - arouses considerable enthusiasm and some outright hostility as well. Its proponents say that nursing specialisms established through custom and usage decades ago have become an anachronism.

'It is possible to make a case for more specialisation, for different specialisms or no specialisation' (p.32).

The argument in favour of a generic nurse is that she would be more widely informed and flexible - especially important in community nursing (DHSS, 1986a). The weight of professional opinion has not however been able to accept a common three year training course. The RCN Commission on Nursing Education was itself divided, but eventually accepted the merits of a common foundation in the first two years' training. This was similarly favoured by the UKCC (1986) which recommended that the three year training contain a branch programme in the final year which entitled the nurse to develop a specialism in: mental handicap, mental illness, midwifery, nursing of adults, and nursing of children. To a degree this replicates the pattern of medical education, but there is little discussion in the UKCC report of the difficulties encountered by medicine in linking individual student choice of specialism with the service's manpower needs. On the community side, both the Cumberlege Report (DHSS, 1986a) and Project 2000, (UKCC, 1986) accept that the main lines of professional division - health visitors, district nurses, community midwives, community psychiatric and community mental handicap nurses - will be retained, although there is a corresponding call for more common training, particularly between health visitors and district nurses.

'We must emphasise that we are not proposing the introduction of a generic nurse, but we do see common training as the one way to break down the rigid roles these nurses have at present' (DHSS, 1986a, p.44).

The current pattern of nurse qualifications contains a further division between enrolled and registered nurse levels. Project 2000 and the ENB Report (1985a) are united in recommending that enrolled nurse training should be ended in favour of one level of nurse. The RCN has been rather less explicit in its support, but it has not been opposed to a development which carries forward part of the recommendations in the Briggs Report (1972) for a single portal of entry, as well as EEC directives which emphasise a three year registration as the basis for a nursing qualification. The justification for change rests largely on the claim that 'nursing is done more efficiently and effectively with only one level of nurse' (UKCC, 1985c). There is scant evidence to support this, suggesting that professional interests are paramount. The enrolled nurse organisations have also been less than enthusiastic about their projected demise, the health unions too expressing their opposition.

An associated issue is the place of 'nursing' auxiliaries and aides. Here the ENB, RCN and UKCC reports present a united front. An assistant level called an aide or helper is recommended. The title 'nurse' is deliberately excluded, although there is a general assumption that these staff will be controlled by nurse managers, and trained locally by nurses, rather than be subject to directives from National Boards. Again professional and manpower issues are likely to come into conflict.

'Those who are anxious to see the demise of the enrolled nurse may not be so willing to see her replaced by an army of auxiliaries, an option which may appeal to the ministers and general managers of this world' (Dickson, 1985, p.28).

The 'army of auxiliaries' looms even larger given the weight of opinion favouring the separation of the service and education sectors in nurse education and training. Project 2000 (UKCC, 1986) recommends that nursing students are given a supernumerary status throughout their training period. This proposal has vast manpower implications for the NHS. It would effectively reduce the nursing workforce by some 85,000 learners, and many hospitals would be seriously threatened because learners provide the majority of direct nursing care to patients. Nevertheless, the UKCC report is adamant that this constitutes 'the single most important move in achieving the requisite level of educational control' (1986, p.84).

This educational argument does not commend itself to all in nursing. There are those who point to the advantages of practical, day-to-day experience in caring for patients as the best method of nurse learning. The upgrading of nurse learners to student status is only part of the professional debate about achieving greater nursing control over the production of new recruits. It widens into a question of where this training should take place. Whereas the Briggs Report (1972) had advocated colleges of nurses and midwifery, and the RCN had made a more ambitious proposal to move into higher education, Project 2000 suggests that the decision is left to the National Boards. Again, the multiple interest groups within a health profession make for difficulties in policy formulation and implementation. At the present time, both the RCN and ENB are in general agreement:

'... that students should be supernumerary (though not for how long), and they have taken similar stances over teacher training. They even agree that nurse training should move into the education sector, although they disagree about how quickly this can be achieved and whether it should include advanced further as well as higher education' (Dickson, 1985, p.28).

The constraints under which these discussions are progressing are much in evidence. Proposals must not cost a lot of money, and they must minimise intraprofessional strife, while also advancing the general professional interest in a wider occupational control and status in the health services. Immediate action is the aim. The UKCC is in a position to introduce new education and training policies by alterations to its existing rules, although some of the changes outlined in Project 2000 will require legislative action. However, its report contains little analysis of the full manpower and cost implications of its proposals as they impact on central and local Health Authorities. To this extent, the professional discussion of nurse production has not taken cognisance of wider manpower debates in the NHS, thus reducing the prospects for significant change.

MANAGEMENT AND NURSE WORKING PRACTICES

The refurbishment of nurse education carries very significant implications for the utilisation of nurses, and vice versa. Equally important is the inter-relationship of nurse education and the nursing career structure. If the medical profession has focussed the management spotlight on problems in its career structure and has minimised external intervention in medical work practices, this does not parallel the experience of nursing. Nurses are currently divided at the point of entry between those who will remain as enrolled nurses, and those others who are eligible for promotion through the nursing grades. However, the pattern of post-Salmon changes in the structure of nursing has been to emphasise the division between those with managerial responsibilities and those who remain at the clinical level. Promotion after the ward sister/charge nurse grade takes the individual into administrative-managerial arenas. Experienced clinical staff are largely withdrawn from direct patient care. Subsequent promotion necessitates completion of a series of management training courses.
The division is exacerbated because nurse managers are in the front line of schemes to

increase the efficient and effective deployment of
staff. NAO (1985b) indicated that this
was an area that had attracted increasing attention
and there is little doubt that working practices in
nursing have been examined more intensively than in
medicine. Areas identified where the utilisation of
nursing staff might be improved covered: nursing
rosters; matching of staff and workload; five day
wards; use of support staff; and comparative
exercises (Part 5). The practice in a shift work
system of having periods of overlap so that staff
can consult about patient care has long been an
accepted feature in the NHS. The Briggs Report
(1972) queried the length of overlap time, and NAO
(1985b) felt that this could be reduced, although it
recognised difficulties in matching patient and
staff days, and in the necessary variation between
wards. There has been further concern that staffing
levels do not always respond as quickly as they
might, for example, to low bed occupancy levels.
Five day wards have also been widely recommended as
a facility for routine and minor surgery. Another
way of ensuring the most efficient utilisation of
nursing resources might be to increase the use of
support staff, so that non-nursing duties could be
delegated. Significant differences in nursing costs
and staff mix ratios in hospitals with generally
similar cases and workload have also encouraged the
development of performance indicators.

This list of possible managerial interventions
is by no means exhaustive. NAO (1985b) was
especially optimistic about the possibilities for
saving money (and reducing the numbers of nurses)
that such exercises would bring. However their
analysis rested almost entirely on the need to cut
costs, and provided no information whatsoever on the
impact of such changes on patient care, let alone
nursing morale. The main criterion seemed to be
that cheapest is best.

The general thrust of the Government to instil
greater concern with efficiency is further
illustrated in the terms of reference for the
review of community nursing services: '... how
resources can be used more effectively, so as to
improve the services available to client groups'
(DHSS, 1986a). This Cumberlege Report offered an
analysis and list of recommendations which
concentrated on professional concerns and interests.
It claimed its policy proposals did not entail:

'... calling for more resources, but a switch of resources within the NHS and better use of existing funds to enable people to have a realistic choice of being cared for at home rather than in hospital or other institution ...' (Foreword).

A close parallel can be seen in the approach taken in Project 2000 where the manpower or cost consequences of its recommendations are not detailed.

Cumberlege identifies 'a chain of weaknesses' in the community nursing services which includes both managerial and professional issues. Unnecessary 'overlap and duplication' in roles is highlighted - both between hospital and community services, and within the latter, between the various groups (not only nurses) who are involved in health related care and support activities. It is even more critical of:

'... the separate, traditional ways of working in which health visitors and district nurses appear to be trapped. It makes teamwork and flexibility of approach difficult if not sometimes impossible' (p.13).

The more effective utilisation of the community workforce is sought through a combination of: more appropriate and common education and training; more flexible working practices; and more integrated team care (ch.3). The report envisages that health visitors, district nurses, school nurses and their support staff will constitute the core of neighbourhood nursing services, but these will be supplemented by specialists such as community midwives, community psychiatric and community mental handicap nurses. Those groups, such as stoma nurses, who are presently based in the hospital service but who are developing a community role, would also be included under community nurse management.

The report also advocates the establishment of primary health care teams - of GPs and nurses - on a formal basis. There should be a written agreement which will specify what nursing support would be provided. GPs who did not negotiate any such arrangement would then only receive those nursing services which the community nurse managers felt able to provide, if any (p.36). The attempt to

generate increased self-management for community
nursing services is further reinforced in the
recommendation that subsidies to GPs who employ
practice nurses should be discontinued (ch.9).
Although this is largely justified on cost grounds,
it also exerts an important appeal for professional
reasons.

There is little disagreement that the
employment of more qualified nurses in the community
will attack spiralling costs where nurses undertake
tasks otherwise provided by doctors (Bowling, 1985a;
1985b; Hart, 1985a, 1985b). Estimates of the number
of practice nurses within the NHS vary: the
Cumberlege Report talks of a rapid growth in numbers
in England between 1974 and 1984 bringing the total
to no more than 4,000 (p.39). Whatever the current
level, all agree that the numbers would at least
treble if GPs took full advantage of the national
scheme which allows for a 70% reimbursement of non-
medical staff salaries (Hart, 1985a, p.1163).

The term 'practice nurse' at present only
signifies that the individual is employed by a GP,
and indicates little about their work tasks. Some
act as nurse-receptionists, while others undertake
procedures which span a wide range of activities
normally associated with the medical role. Studies
have, for example, recorded practice nurses
monitoring blood pressure, counselling, conducting
cervical smears, immunisations, vaccinations and
injections (Bowling, 1985b). The DHSS has declined
to intervene so as to specify exactly what tasks
might properly be delegated to a nurse. For its
part, the medical profession has been unsure how far
the advantages of delegating 'routine' work,
including that for which the doctor can claim an
item-of-service payment such as vaccinations,
outweigh the threat of nurses taking over some areas
at least of general practice. Bowling's (1981)
research concluded that most GPs adopt a fairly
cautious approach with as many as three quarters in
her study practising little or no task delegation.

The nursing profession has generally favoured
an enhanced role for qualified staff insofar as this
pays due recognition to nursing's particular
contribution and skills. In general practice this
means an emphasis on a health preventive and
promotional role rather than a 'cure' oriented model
(Bowling, 1985a; Fullard et al, 1984). This
expansion into health prevention and promotion
accords fully with the philosophy underlying the

91

Cumberlege Report. Even so, not all the profession are so enthusiastic. The RCN has not elaborated what tasks might be suitable for delegation to nurses - whether employed by a GP or a Health Authority. Instead it prefers to emphasise those tasks which signify nursing's independent professional contribution to health care rather than expand into routine or trivial medical procedures (Bowling, 1985b).

The most 'extended' role currently advocated among nurses is that of the nurse practitioner (Stilwell, 1982a; 1984). Again, the training and qualifications, work content and responsibilities have not been the subject of DHSS or professional guidelines. The reaction within nursing circles has been mixed, although the Cumberlege Report endorsed their growth in the community services (DHSS, 1986a, ch.7). A nurse practitioner would then constitute part of the nursing service 'offered' to GPs' practices. The nurse practitioner would provide an alternative, first point of contact with patients, as well as developing a range of preventive and health promotional programmes. There is however little examination of the planning and production of nurse practitioners, and issues of their utilisation in health care are not confronted. Instead the Cumberlege Report dwells on professional unease that the development of a new nursing role in the community will intensify existing conflicts over who (health visitor, district nurse, midwife, etc) does what. In contrast, the recommendation to grant prescribing powers to community nurses offers the possiblity of an enhanced nurse role as well as more efficient working practices without stimulating intra-professional rivalries. The issues of practice nurses and an enlargement in their role are explored further in Chapter 11 below.

It is significant that the examination of nurse manpower management focusses almost exclusively on relations with the medical profession. 'Team care' is a matter for doctors and nurses alone, and 'substitution' raises questions about what medical tasks might be better undertaken by nursing personnel. Allied health professionals have little place on the manpower agenda within nursing. There are some exceptions. For example, Newson (1982) assessed the involvement of physiotherapists rather than midwives giving instructions on physical exercise to pregnant women. The midwives argued that this lowered the effectiveness and continuity of ante-natal care, and not least their own occupational control. In contrast, a team based approach as usually interpreted by nurses spotlights the opportunities to extend the nursing role and diminish medical dominance.

INTEGRATING THE MANPOWER PROCESS

The discussion in earlier sections has emphasised that the development of the nurse manpower process has been uneven, although at times highly regarded for its technical sophistication. As with other health care practitioners, problems have been experienced in balancing national and local interests, just as nurse manpower policies provide further evidence of continuing struggles over occupational control and status. In contrast to medicine, nursing does not enjoy anything like the same 'unmanaged' status. The manpower process in nursing diverges in other respects. Most distinctly, a greater proportion of the planning, production and management of nurse manpower is conducted at the local level. This is reinforced in the organisational structures and arrangements. The central Health Departments have adopted a high profile in aspects of the manpower process, but they do not exercise a policy making role comparable with that for medical manpower. For example, there is not the same involvement in national demand and supply forecasting. Nor is the central control of hospital physician posts matched by equivalent action for nurses.

Central Health Departments, professional manpower bodies and consultative procedures that abound for physicians have far fewer equivalents in the numerically much larger and as diversified nursing profession. The wider scope for local action has meant that the primary focus for integrating nurse manpower policies has been the translation of local Health Authority interventions to the ward, unit or community levels. The national level plays less of a control role than in medicine, acting rather more in an advisory and facilitative manner. Nevertheless, as the growth of demand methodologies has mushroomed, the effect of local nurse managers and manpower planners devising their own approaches has been both to satisfy higher level Authorities that a more efficient and effective use of resources is being implemented and to convince clinical staff that these are acceptable in regard to patient care. Although this may make

the manpower process less visible to central Health
Departments, it merely translates the inherent
problems of integrating nurse manpower policies to a
lower level in the organisational and planning
system.

The central pressures to enhance the manpower
process illustrates the specific political context
in which nursing is located. The engagement with
manpower issues has presented important challenges
in its struggle to achieve full professional status,
and the degree of autonomous authority in its
occupational practice which that implies. Yet the
pressures to generate particular manpower policies,
if they cannot easily be ignored in the NHS, might
also be the means for enhanced nurse management of
its affairs. The discussion of nursing supply and
demand indicates how nurses have been swayed by
economic and manpower controls in devising
'objective' measures, but also how this has provided
some opportunities to legitimise the role of
professional judgement. Indeed, the professional
contribution has increasingly sought to direct these
manpower debates into areas which give greater
weight to quality of care as evaluated by nurses
themselves. Together with developments on the
general management front, political and professional
isolation is a continuing theme which means that the
integration of the nurse manpower process holds the
prospect of significant conflicts at the local
level.

Chapter 6

ALLIED HEALTH PROFESSIONALS

While medical and nursing staff are frequently the
subject of manpower examination, there are
significant numbers of other practitioners who have
a close involvement in patient care and whose
contribution to the delivery of health services
warrants more detailed investigation. The umbrella
term of 'allied health professionals' (AHPs)
indicates a general reference point. Most NHS
commentators have highlighted the form of these
practitioners' relationship with physicians,
although the extent of any dependence and overlap
varies. The widening choice of labels for these
staff - 'paramedical', 'supplementary', 'allied', or
'complementary' professions - indicates the
problematic character of their work and
organisational positions (Stocking, 1979). The
general references to 'allied health professionals'
should not though be allowed to mask the
considerable variation in their occupational control
and status.

The concentration of allied health
professionals is in the 'Professional and Technical
Staff' (P and T) and 'Other Practitioner' categories
identified by the central Health Departments (see
Chapter 3, Table 3.1). P and T itself spans over
thirty different staff groups. The most referenced
are the professions operating under the Council for
Professions Supplementary to Medicine (CPSM), that
is, chiropodists, dieticians, medical laboratory
scientific officers (formerly technicians),
occupational therapists, physiotherapists,
radiographers and remedial gymnasts. The latter
group is in the midst of an amalgamation with the
physiotherapists. Speech therapists are widely
linked with these 'remedial' professions, although
not actually included in the Professions
Supplementary to Medicine Act (PSM Act) of 1960. In
addition to this PSM group and associated aides and
helpers, P and T embraces highly qualified
scientific staff, such as biochemists, physicists

and psychologists, together with hospital pharmacists and opticians, and a range of technicians, including dental surgery assistants, pharmacy, medical and dark room technicians, who possess basic educational qualifications and undergo only minimal professional training. The remainder of the AHP staff are categorised as 'Other Practitioners', who unlike the P and T group are located in the Family Practitioner Services. These comprise pharmacists, opticians and opthalmic medical practitioners. Only occasional reference will be made in the following discussion to their situation.

This Chapter explores the development of the health manpower process across these staff groups. A breakdown of manpower in the AHP group is presented in Table 6.1. It is argued that the consideration of the manpower issues is generally less sophisticated technically, and typically accorded a lower priority by Health Authorities than is the case with either physicians or nurses. The relatively small number of staff in many of the occupational groups, coupled with their wide dispersal across Health Authorities, and the relatively moderate impact of AHPs on health expenditure, have all played their part in inhibiting manpower discussions.

PLANNING ALLIED HEALTH PROFESSIONS

The PSM Act established registration boards for the professions operating under the CPSM. Each board was given responsibilities for education and training, and for maintaining registers of qualified personnel. Although not covered by the Act, similar regulations apply to speech therapists. More widely, pharmacy is covered by legislation which requires registration with the appropriate professional association - the Pharmaceutical Society.

However, while the CPSM and the boards it supervises exercise important powers in respect of those wishing to work in the NHS, they cannot prevent unregistered (unqualified) individuals practising in private employment outside the NHS as, for example, chiropodists or physiotherapists. These professions can restrict use of titles such as 'state registered' or 'registered', but they do not have exclusive claim to the designation as a 'chiropodist' or 'physiotherapist'.

The Royal Commission on the NHS Report (1979,

Table 6.1: Allied Health Professionals in England,
Scotland and Wales, 30 September, 1983
(Whole Time Equivalents)

	England	Scotland	Wales
Chiropodists	2,392	435	156
Dieticians	819	160	46
Occupational Therapists	3,377	371	145
Orthoptists	444	43	23
Physiotherapists	7,719	1,033*	424
Radiographers	7,576	909	507
Remedial Gymnasts	372	*	42
Helpers/Aides (for OTs, Physios & Radiographers)	6,259	322	362
Speech Therapists	1,973	308	92
Medical Laboratory Scientific Officers	14,718	2,193	885
Scientists & Psychologists	3,866	533	204
Technicians	14,312	2,450	1,836
Hospital Pharmacists & Opticians	3,329	487	227**
Other Professional & Technical Staff	1,715	246	97

Source: DHSS, Health and Personal Social Service
Statistics for England 1985, Table 3.14;
Welsh Office, Health and Personal Social
Service Statistics for Wales 1985, Table
3.17; and Common Services Agency for the
Scottish Health Authority (1986), Scottish
Health Statistics 1984, Tables 9.1 and 9.2.

Key: *   Physiotherapists and remedial gymnasts
combined in Scotland.
**   No figures available for hospital opticians
in Wales.

Chapter 15) expressed some concern that the PSM were becoming too rigid in their staffing policies and called for a review of manpower planning across these groups. The CPSM for its part argued that it should take on a manpower planning role since there was little central guidance on the number and type of professional skills required. Although some such planning effort was made in the late 1970s, that ambition has now been rejected by central government.

Estimates of the demand for AHPs have rarely extended beyond staffing norms. For example, Remedial Therapist (December 1984, p.1) talked of a shortfall in occupational therapists (OTs) of some 2,000 which implied that the total number of OTs in the NHS needed to double. The Chartered Society of Physiotherapy has attempted to provide a fairly detailed breakdown of staff-per-bed ratios. These range from 1:5 in an intensive care situation, through 1:15 where physiotherapists are utilised as part of an intensive programme of assessment and rehabilitation, down to 1:120 in short stay obstetric units and in long stay maintenance wards with geriatric and psycho-geriatric beds.

The demand for AHPs is expected to expand, especially with the increasing percentage of elderly in the population, and the growing proportion of frail elderly who have greater health care needs for such groups as chiropodists, physiotherapists and dieticians. Between 1974 and 1977 there was, for example, a 20% increase in the number of treatments provided by chiropodists, and over 90% of patients receiving these services were aged 65 years or more (Royal Commission on the NHS, Report, 1979, para.8.23). But although such demographic and epidemiological factors affect the demand for AHPs, there have been few attempts to trace through this relationship.

'The growing demands for services related to the physically and mentally handicapped, the mentally ill and the elderly, as well as the extension of the physiotherapist's role in occupational health and in health education, are recognised but largely unmet, due to lack of funds or problems of recruitment' (Chartered Society of Physiotherapy, 1986, p.80).

Although all of the AHPs recount a similar tale of expanding manpower needs, it is rarely supported with detailed research material. There is evidence of considerable variation between local Health Authorities in their employment of AHPs, which may reflect the attractiveness of employment in different areas as much as deliberate policy.

The historical development of services mostly has its basis in medical referral. For example, the GP as the first point of contact for health care is usually responsible for initiating remedial care, and is in a position to significantly inflate or diminish demand for such treatment. The Seebohm Report of 1968 concluded that there was a considerable ignorance among GPs of rehabilitation services, and subsequent research has indicated how widely physicians vary in their readiness to refer disabled patients, for example, to occupational therapy. Busuttil's (1985) research suggested that the variation in physician response was based sometimes on ignorance of what services were available, and sometimes on a lack of conviction as to their effectiveness.

In 1975 the Halsbury Report (1975, para.60 ff) noted that while there 'are no nationally recognised standards of staffing' and 'the figures must be treated with caution, as staffing standards vary and the scale of need is bound to some extent to be impressionistic', there was evidence of significant staff shortages: for example, 55% in occupational therapy, 50% in dietetics, 35% in physiotherapy, 25% in radiography, and 20% in orthoptics (para.63). Subsequent experience has been that employment prospects in several groups, especially among the newly qualified, have been much less assured. Thus although demand is still felt to outdistance supply, the lack of government funding, or its translation in employment opportunities at the local level, has become the major factor in determining manpower requirements.

The restriction on NHS finance is highlighted as the major factor of demand in Stocking's (1979) wide-ranging review of the 'complementary' professions in the NHS. Changes in resource availability have easily overridden other indicators of need. They may well also constrain other indicators of priority since it is likely to be organisationally simpler to 'freeze' unfilled vacancies in designated areas than to run down existing staff levels in sectors of lesser importance in order to release finance to fill the staff vacancy.

On the supply side, all of the labour market factors widely referenced for health care are relevant, although it is not clear how important relative levels of pay are in aiding recruitment. Given the predominance of females in these professions, together with the considerable extent of part-time employment in some of them, social changes concerning family timing and continued employment after childbirth may be expected to be important determinants of supply. Also important is the extent to which there exist opportunities for employment outside the NHS. For example, in occupational therapy employment by local authority social services is possible at more attractive rates of pay. Such opportunities exist for most of the relevant professions, but are in most cases restricted to the relatively small number of private health care organisations operating in Britain. A few professions however, notably chiropody and pharmacy, have much greater opportunities for private practice. For example, according to the Report of the Royal Commission on the National Health Service:

> 'There are about 5,000 chiropodists on the register (of the Society of Chiropodists) but only about two-thirds of those work for the NHS .... There are, therefore, a substantial number of chiropodists who would be eligible for NHS employment but who work only in private practice. In addition, there is an unknown number, possibly amounting to several thousands, of people who practise some chiropody, perhaps on a part-time basis, and are not registered. The NHS is competing for registered chiropodists with the attractions of independent private practice' (1979, para. 8.25).

Of equal importance on the supply side is the impact of agencies involved in the production of these professions. For example, the qualifications recognised for state registration of radiographers, occupational therapists, physiotherapists, remedial gymnasts, orthoptists, and chiropodists are diplomas issued by the appropriate professional body, which in all the above cases also effectively operates as the trade union for the profession. Since the qualifying role gives a degree of control over the schools where the qualification is pursued, it also gives a significant control over the maximum numbers of persons trained each year, which is quite independent of the NHS's planning or management

arrangements. This power has not been employed as
much as it might have been, though the College of
Radiographers reduced the number of training places
by one-third in 1978 in response to fears of
unemployment (Harrison, 1981). The Royal Commission
on the National Health Service (Report, 1979,
paras.8.26 and 15.6) suggested that chiropodists
might be seeking to limit entry unreasonably - an
allegation which has not been substantiated (CPSM,
1980a, p.4). Linstead (1984) has extended this type
of analysis to physiological measurement
technicians, a group not covered by state
registration arrangements. Attempts at manpower
planning in one Region have been vitiated by the
unwillingness of educational institutions to support
proposals which might result in the reallocation of
students amongst institutions, and of heads of
technical departments to switch from a weekly day
release system of education to one of block release,
involving the student in long absences from the
workplace.
    Unlike for the medical profession there have
been relatively few attempts to model the stocks and
flows of the AHPs, and most of the work which has
taken place has been both partial and undertaken by
the professional bodies rather than by government,
managers or planners. The only official attempt to
undertake such analysis was carried out by the DHSS
(1980b and 1981c) in respect of occupational
therapists, chiropodists, physiotherapists and
radiographers. More recently, central government
attention has shifted towards controlling the
numbers of non-direct patient care staff, with a
consequent reduction of interest in manpower
planning. Some NHS Regions conducted their own
attempts to model professional manpower at subnational level (Harrison and Brooks, 1985). In
addition, a very small number of academic studies
have been conducted, such as Jack and Alpine's
(1980) study of opticians. Another relevant report
is that of the Society of Radiographers which as
noted above led to a reduction of student numbers,
which has remained in force notwithstanding its
formally temporary character. A joint survey by the
Pharmaceutical Society and the University Grants
Committee in 1978 led to the conclusion that intake
to pharmacy courses should be reduced (Stocking,
1979, p.100). More recent professional comment has
focussed on the supply problems for hospital
pharmacists. Other studies which have been carried
out have sought to establish staffing norms, for

instance in respect of occupational therapists
(based on staff-patient ratios: College of
Occupational Therapists, 1980) and pharmacists
(based on patient data as a proxy for workload:
Briggs et al, 1980). Finally, the Association of
Chief Chiropody Officers carried out a survey in
1980, aimed at identifying for the first time a
range of basic information about manpower resources
employed within that profession.

PRODUCTION: EDUCATION AND TRAINING

In contrast to the relative dearth of material
concerning the estimation of the demand for and
supply of allied health professions, there is a much
more voluminous and detailed literature, especially
emanating from the professions themselves, on
recruitment, education and training. This is not
surprising because the PSM boards are charged with
responsibilities in this area and to a lesser degree
manpower management, rather than manpower planning.
These boards, one for each profession and with a
majority of their membership elected directly from
that profession, are responsible for state
registration, including the recognition of
registrable qualifications. The thrust of this body
of literature concerning production and professional
roles can be summarised under four headings:
training; education and academic standards;
regulation; and autonomy. These are dealt with in
turn below.

It is apparent that the allied health
professionals are intent on trying to improve the
extent of their occupational control. A key area
has been enhanced professional regulation of
recruitment and training. The system among AHPs is
however very complex and involves local, regional
and central Health and Education Departments, as
well as the professional societies themselves. This
multi-institional arrangement takes a number of
forms. For example, physiotherapy and remedial
gymnastics students are mainly funded by DHSS
bursaries, although the latter are on NHS salaries
for the practical year. Chiropody students in
contrast are mostly supported by LEA grants, with
relatively little NHS sponsorship (Harrison and
Brooks, 1985). These largely reflect different
training arrangements:

'Most orthoptists, physiotherapists,
radiographers and remedial gymnasts are trained

at NHS based schools; but most occupational
therapy (and speech therapy) schools are
outside the NHS, though making use of the NHS
for practical work; while dieticians take a
polytechnic or university course. There are
three NHS chiropody schools, the rest of those
training to registration standard being in
colleges of further education' (Royal
Commission Report, 1979, para.15.10).

The training system for PSM is therefore extremely
diverse but the opportunities for non-professional
bodies to influence the production of staff exist in
all areas, although these appear to have been
exploited sparingly (Stocking, 1979, pp.88-91).
Obviously a transfer of a training school from a
private or NHS setting to the higher education arena
(or vice versa) has potentially important
consequences for the funding and general control of
professional training and employment opportunities.
There has also been a call for a shift to DES
funding, for example, of physiotherapists (Williams,
1984).
    A second thrust of the literature relates to
higher academic standards, both for recruitment to
education for the professions and in respect of the
professional qualification itself. The PSM group
have argued that the level of professional
qualification should be changed from Diploma to
Degree level, thus raising their status to that of
graduate professions such as pharmacy. Some of
these professions are already committed to a shift
towards all-graduate qualification, including
occupational therapy, chiropody (CPSM, 1981, pp.5-
7), physiotherapy (Harrison and Brooks, 1985), and
dietetics (Stocking, 1979, p.110), but others have
proceeded more cautiously to suggest a partial
shift, perhaps with a two-tier profession of
registered and enrolled grades (CPSM, 1977,
pp.7-20). Related to this call are the trends,
already occurring, for the schools for these
professions to move from the NHS into the Further
Education sector (p.4), for the qualification
courses to be lengthened to three years (CPSM, 1981,
p.8), and for General Certificate of Education at
Advanced Level to be required for entry to training
(Stocking, 1979, p.110). These changes have often
been explained in relation to the need to establish
a research base for the professions (SHHD, 1984).
    Thirdly, the PSM group is regulated to the
extent that state registration is required before

employment can be obtained in the profession within the NHS. However, the CPSM, after extensive consultations within the professions, has recently suggested a number of changes in relevant legislation which would have the effect of considerably increasing the present degree of regulation. There are two major recommendations (CPSM, 1980b). At present, employment in the NHS in the eight occupations covered by the CPSM is restricted to the state-registered, but an extension to this restriction is being sought in order to prevent the use of the title of the profession ('physiotherapist' and so on) to the non-state-registered. This would have the effect of curtailing the activities of non-registered persons in the private sector. Current indications are that the government is in some sympathy with a change of this kind or with similar effect. The other extension is the power to require professionals periodically to demonstrate their continued competency, by either approved experience or by a test, in order to retain state registration. It is worth noting that a parallel trend of tighter regulation is discernible within the nursing profession, in respect of health visitors, occupational health nurses and midwives (Stocking, 1979, p.109).

Fourthly, the literature reflects a trend towards more autonomy within these professions. As Stocking (1979, p.114) notes, the different professions show considerable variations in the degree of autonomy of their practice, particularly in regard to whether patients can be referred directly or only via a physician, and the extent to which the nature of the treatment to be given is specified by a referring physician. Following the recommendations of the <u>McMillan Report</u> (DHSS, 1973), the DHSS and the medical profession agreed that the doctor should retain overall responsibility for patient care, while no longer attempting to specify the precise form which occupational therapy, physiotherapy and remedial gymnastic treatment should take (Health Circular HC(77)33). According to Ovretveit (1985, p.88), one result has been that:

'The history of the development of professional autonomy in physiotherapy ... shows that there has been a decline in certain aspects of medical dominance over the profession, but the medical profession retains important elements of control'.

Stocking (1979, p.121) notes the same trend in the profession of clinical psychology, members of which have sought the right to treat patients independently of physicians. The desire to obtain equal status with the medically qualified consultant is discernible in some other scientific professions, such as biochemistry.

There have also been calls to speed up the creation of unqualified 'aides' to many of these professions, such as foot hygienists who undertake basic foot care tasks under the direction of a registered chiropodist. In 1977 such persons totalled less than 30 whole time equivalents in the UK (Royal Commission Report, para.8.27, Table 15.1). The College of Occupational Therapists has similarly sought the expansion of 'helpers'; training courses are provided in a number of Regions (Mead et al, 1985). The development of unqualified helpers is nevertheless regarded with misgivings in some quarters lest the aide's role is extended in ways which diminish professional control. This unease has been well-documented among radiographers who argue that only those with the appropriate scientific training should use x-rays (Stocking, 1979, p.136).

A further strand in this autonomy literature with a potential impact on production is the extent to which the professions should widen their role to undertake independent clinical assessments. The potential for conflict with physicians, in particular, and also nurses, is a source of concern within the NHS. Examples of such changes include the claims for clinical psychologists to be solely responsible for techniques of behaviour modification (ibid, p.121), of physiotherapists to be responsible for acupuncture, for chiropodists to undertake foot surgery (CPSM, 1983a) and to be less restricted in their employment of analgesics, and for radiographers to expand their involvement in new technologies such as CT scanning, ultrasound, and Nuclear Magnetic Resonance (SHHD, 1984, p.38).

The production aspect of the manpower process demonstrates a considerable range of issues, and large variation among the constituent groups of allied health professionals. There is widespread concern among AHPs that insufficient control is exercised by the professional groups, although the perceived difficulties and the proposed solutions do not offer a common pattern.

MANAGEMENT ISSUES

The literature on the most efficient and effective utilisation of the allied health professional workforce is again extremely sparse, and limited in its management perspective. The sole areas of debate revolve around fears over the lack of 'self-management' in these groups, and some discussion of a more appropriate career structure. The overwhelming impression is of the ways in which issues of manpower management are perceived as threats to groups who already consider that their professional status is not generally accepted in the NHS.

Thus, in addition to the movement towards greater clinical autonomy, steps have been taken towards what Mercer (1981) terms 'administrative autonomy', that is the opportunity for the professions to be self-managing. It is possible that the pursuit of additional administrative autonomy is an alternative strategy to the pursuit of additional clinical autonomy. Amongst the several manifestations of this trend have been the creation of managerial hierarchies within each profession and a series of disputes between the professions and other actors. These have included arguments over the merits of appointing managers of individual paramedical services at District (multi-institution) level (Williams et al, 1981; Donald, 1981), over whether the involvement of such managers in the formal mechanisms of management have had any impact upon their ability to influence matters (Harrison and Henly, 1982), and over whether pathology laboratories should be managed by physicians, scientists or technicians (Royal Commission Report, 1979).

The opinion that, as in nursing, recent initiatives to enhance and refurbish NHS management both threaten the health professions in general, and fail to recognise important differences between them has been widely articulated. At the present time there is considerable variation in the management of AHPs. Table 6.2 depicts the range of professional autonomy and management practices within the PSM group and speech therapists.

Table 6.2: Aspects of Management Structure and
Clinical Practice among Selected Allied Health
Professionals

<u>PROFESSIONAL AUTONOMY</u> *   <u>MANAGEMENT</u> **

CHIROPODISTS

Independent practitioners   Profession substantially
 - medical referral   engaged in private
possible, but not   practice. Within NHS,
required. Treatment to   hierarchical management
be confined to   structure up to District
'maintenance of the feet   level.
in a healthy condition
and the treatment of
their disabilities by
recognised chiropodial
methods in which the
practitioner has been
trained'. Occasional
friction with medical
profession over practice
of podiatry.

DIETICIANS

Independent practitioners   Hierarchical management
but they may not   structure up to District
'habitually treat ...   level; not universally
any individual patient   implemented.
therapeutically without
instructions given by a
registered medical or
dental practitioner'.

MEDICAL LABORATORY OFFICERS
SCIENTIFIC OFFICERS (MLSOs)

May not seek to   Hierarchical management
diagnose or treat   structure within
disease. With the   laboratories, and
exception of pregnancy   sometimes up to District
testing, may not report   level. Some tension over
on any specimen unless   management role of
'the diagnosis and/or   pathologists (physicians)
treatment are to be   and biochemists in
performed by a registered   relation to MLSOs and
medical (or) dental ...   overall laboratory
practitioner.'   management.

OCCUPATIONAL THERAPISTS

May only work on referral from a registered medical practitioner unless the therapist has 'direct access to the patient's doctor'. Some pressure for more independent practice.

Co-ordinating and advising role of District OT exists, not totally implemented. Not strictly an executive role.

ORTHOPTISTS

Work only on referral from a physician, except where part of a 'screening procedure or assessment programme' approved by a physician.

Hierachical structure within profession within departments. No District level post, and generally included in Opthalmic Department.

PHYSIOTHERAPISTS ***

Must confine work to fields for which trained, and should not treat unless the patient 'has been referred ... by a registered medical or dental practitioner, except in an emergency or for some other exceptional reason or unless he/she has direct access to the patient's doctor'. More independent clinical practice is actively being sought by the profession, and referring physicians rarely now specify the nature of the treatment required.

Co-ordinating and advisory role of District Physiotherapist exists. Not strictly an executive role.

RADIOGRAPHERS

May not purport to diagnose injury or disease except, in the

Hierarchical structure within departments and sometimes up to District absence of a radiologist; may orally communicate the appearance of an x-ray to the physician in charge of the case. May only accept patients for examination or treatment on referral from a registered medical or dental practitioner.

level. Some tension over radiologist's (physician's) management role in relation to radiotherapy and x-ray generally.

REMEDIAL GYMNASTS ***

May only work on referral from a physician

Too small to have a management structure

SPEECH THERAPISTS

No formal state registration required though NHS may only employ persons holding certificate of College of Speech Therapy. May work on referral from physician, health visitor, teacher (etc), or on self-referral.

Management structure up District level.

Source: Stocking, 1979, Table 1, adapted.

* Comments in quotation marks are from the relevant statements of conduct governing discipline in the profession, and were current at 31 March 1986.

** Management arrangements are as at the date of fieldwork. Since then, the implementation of the Griffiths Report (DHSS, 1983c) has called functional management arrangements (in these and other occupations) into serious question, and at the time of writing these are beginning to break down.

*** The professions of physiotherapy and remedial gymnasts merged in 1985/86.

A further illustration of the issues at stake in manpower management is provided by recent discussions of management budgeting and costing. For example, a district physiotherapist has charged management consultants with total disregard for physiotherapy's specific area of practice by treating it as if it were:

'a functional service similar to pharmacy or radiography, with a product which could be ordered by a doctor and charged directly to a user-budget. There have even been attempts to develop standard cost units using time as a base.... The introduction of these systems will turn back the clock on a profession which has won its professional freedom after a long struggle. It is therefore bound to be somewhat sensitive to measures which fail to recognise the nature of physiotherapy practice' (Williams, 1985, p.1128).

In the context of professionalisation and increasing economic and manpower controls, physiotherapists have tried to gain acceptance as a clinical budget holder. In a similar fashion, physiotherapists have disputed proposals from the Korner Steering Group on health services information that the number of patients seen should be the criterion of work done as this ignores all activities beyond the therapeutic role (ibid, p.1129).

The Chartered Society of Physiotherapy has argued for an extension and strengthening of district physiotherapy management rather than of general management. The rationale offered is that

'physiotherapy is a cross-medical specialty and a cross-unit service .... While accepting the need for administrative accountability to more senior management, physiotherapists cannot accept professional accountability to general managers, doctors, or anyone other than a member of their own profession. This professional accountability cannot be divorced from the control of the resources used to achieve the effective treatment of patients' (CSP, 1984).

In physiotherapy, as in the other PSM, there has been an appreciation that arguments for professional control over manpower need to be phrased in terms of cost effectiveness and efficiency (Williams et al, 1981). There remains little research evidence to back up claims on either side. Evaluative studies of the quality of care concentrate on particular therapeutic interventions within a specific professional area. There is almost no work on the comparative contribution of, say, occupational therapy and physiotherapy in the care of the elderly, nor is there any detailed review of the efficacy of multi-disciplinary teams. Most discussion in the literature concentrates on the independent clinical contribution rather than the possibilities of an approach rooted in team care.

CONCLUSION

On the basis of the literature reviewed, three main observations are worthy of emphasis. Firstly, the responsibility for making major decisions concerning both the numbers and the roles of these professions is fragmented amongst a large number of institutions, many of which are not under the managerial control of the NHS. Secondly, decisions are taken in reaction to immediately perceived problems rather than on a more strategic basis. Many of the most recent attempts to look at manpower are spurred by the need to make financial savings and have resulted in a range of somewhat crude and sometimes perverse manpower policies. Thirdly, there has been little attempt to look beyond the existing division of labour; decisions and arguments have largely reflected professional self-interest or at least a somewhat narrow point of view. It can thus be seen that the manpower process for the professions discussed is far from well-integrated into the planning of services or of capital projects, and shows little sign of immediately becoming so.

Chapter 7

A SURVEY OF MANPOWER PRACTICES

INTRODUCTION

This Chapter presents findings from an interview
based survey of a small number of Health Authorities
and from a postal questionnaire survey sent to one
in three Authorities within England and Wales. Its
purpose is to outline the state and range of current
practices in health manpower, exploring in
particular the planning and management dimensions
and also the production side, as well as mechanisms
for and constraints to their integration. Its focus
lies solely on manpower practices within the field
of activity of District Health Authorities and thus
excludes concern with the primary health care
context.
 The interview based survey was carried out in
April to October 1984 with the objectives of
clarifying areas of concern to actors in the
manpower field and of ensuring that the issues
raised in the questionnaire were intelligible and
relevant. The intention was therefore to use the
interviews as a pilot for the postal questionnaire
survey, as well as a means of generating detailed
information on manpower practices in the areas
studied. In all, interviews took place in 15
Authorities, both Regional and District, and lasted
about one to two hours each. They were administered
to 32 individuals ranging from personnel officers,
unit administrators, and medical, nursing and
paramedical heads of departments. Choice of
individuals and Health Authorities to explore was
guided by advice received from Regional Manpower
Planning specialists as to 'places of particular
interest' or 'places developing expertise in the
field'. Topic areas explored are outlined in Table
7.1, each being addressed in an open-ended manner,
allowing the pursuit of relevant lines of enquiry as
they emerged in the interview.

Table 7.1: Areas Investigated in the Semi-Structured Interviews

A Contextual Issues

   . What are the financial and other constraints
     on manpower planning at this level in the
     organisation?
   . What is the general approach to planning
     ('top-down' vs 'bottom-up')?

B Respondent's Role in Manpower Planning

   . How are the number of staff required
     identified (norms vs demand vs needs-based;
     and if norms, their sources)?
   . Is manpower planned by staff group (nurse,
     physician, etc) or client care groups
     (elderly, mentally ill, etc)?
   . What consideration is given to skill mix
     roles, etc?
   . If a new/another physician is to be appointed,
     are non-physician manpower implications
     thought through?

D Manpower Supply

   . What information exists on potential source
     of supply, manpower stock, labour market,
     register of former nurses?
   . What influences are there over local training
     facilities and sources of recruitment
     (internal and external), and how extensive are
     they?
   . If a key person cannot be recruited, what
     then? Is substitution and role enlargement
     possible and acceptable?
   . To what extent can the Health Authority
     influence supply?
   . Are there any specific policies on encouraging
     women to return to work (creches, flexibility
     of hours)?

E Implementation

   . Who is responsible for the implementation of
     the manpower content of the plan? What
     measures are there to ensure implementation?

Building on this pilot interview survey in order to generate a representative range of health manpower practices, a postal questionnaire was drawn up (see Appendix) and circulated in November 1984 to one in three District Health Authorities in England and Wales. Scotland and Northern Ireland were excluded from the study due to pressures of time and limitations of resources. Areas explored in the questionnaire embraced the way manpower requirements were established, strategies used to ensure that required manpower was achieved, whether manpower was planned on a staff group basis or on the lines of a multi-disciplinary team, the general context surrounding manpower planning, and the respondent's own role in the manpower process.

Questionnaires were sent to four groups of persons at the District and Unit level:

1 District Personnel Officers (DPOs), who have a broad ranging responsiblity for the health manpower process;
2 Chief Nursing Officers (CNO) and Directors of Nursing Services (DNS) for the Elderly and for the Community (the DNS were chosen because of their contrasting role with the CNO and the specific primary health care relevance of their respective client groups);
3 The District Head Physiotherapist and District Occupational Therapist, representing two of the allied health professionals; and
4 District Medical Officers, in their role as medical advisor to the Health Authority.

Sampling was constructed to obtain representativeness of teaching and non-teaching Districts, those with and without an occupational therapy or physiotherapy training school, urban and rural Health Authorities, and locations with higher proportions of over-65 year olds or not. An overall response rate of 57% was achieved. Actual response rates varied by professional group; that is, personnel (34%), nursing (50%), occupational therapists (71%), physiotherapists (64%), and medical officers (78%).

The questionnaire sent in January 1985 to the District Medical Officer in each of the sampled Health Authorities was in the form of a short letter. Two questions were asked. Firstly, how is a decision reached on the need for a new consultant post and, in particular, what criteria are employed, who initiates the process, and how approval for the creation of the post is obtained? Secondly, how is a decision reached to create a new junior medical staff post and what are the policies on the required ratios between junior and consultant staff? It should be pointed out that the responses varied greatly in the amount of detail provided. The findings presented below indicate the range of approaches and highlight noteworthy instances of District level medical manpower planning in practice.

MANPOWER MANAGEMENT DIMENSION

Prior to the undertaking of any survey work, the strategic plans drawn up by the 14 English Regional Health Authorities arising from the 1978-79 strategic planning round were perused, to examine the attention given to manpower, and to ask in the fieldwork how far these plans had been implemented. The documents, the then most current strategic plans, covered the period 1979-88. The subsequent strategic planning round, due to various turns of events, was occurring during the timescale of the study. Strategic plans were not produced by Districts and Regions until after the study was completed; these covered the years 1985-1994. It remains to be seen the extent to which such plans are implemented, and the amount of attention given to manpower within them.

Several comments can be made on the 1979-88 plans. Firstly, an initial assessment of the plans suggested wide divergence in terms of policies and service provision between Regions gaining resources and those losing them under the 'RAWP' allocations. In the RAWP gaining Authorities, an expansion of preventive and primary services was advocated, together with services for the elderly, the mentally ill and the handicapped, in line with government priorities. In the RAWP losing Authorities, in contrast, protection of acute services was argued for as a primary objective. However, upon closer analysis this apparent division became more diffuse, with the policies containing more similarities than differences. For example, in the RAWP gaining Regions whilst they indicated the need for an increase in manpower and capital expenditure on primary care and geriatrics, they also argued for the expansion of acute services and associated manpower, especially in consultant medical and professional staff. Further, in the RAWP losing

Regions, in principle an expansion of resources for PHC was advocated but at the same time the general feeling was that '... resources are locked into existing acute services and cannot be switched'. In addition in some Regions such an argument was justified by reference to:

> 'the lack of primary care services and the need for extra care of the elderly; there is a high useage of acute services by the elderly, and where primary care is inadequate, the demand on secondary care becomes greater' (A Regional Plan 1979-88).

Secondly, turning away from service objectives to manpower, the plans were in general extremely vague about manpower requirements and their achievement. Little analysis or discussion of manpower strategies is apparent, or how any manpower plan was to be implemented. Several Regions failed to acknowledge the existence of staff other than medical consultants and nurses; the remainder were grouped under the heading of 'other'. A concern with creating an information base was often mentioned, mostly as an explanation for the lack of detailed staff breakdown and analyses.

Thirdly, as to the supply of labour, little assessment was given. The general approach tended to be to react to a potential shortage of staff by opening a training school, often with no attention to the available pool of labour to take up resulting places. Further, little, if any, consideration was given to the causes of any shortage of staff. Where this was explored, the cause was usually seen as external - for example, the 'good local employment conditions outside of the NHS'. The possibilities of greater resort to part-time openings, refresher courses and other flexible arrangements for the predominantly female labour force were not mentioned. Finally, there was a tendency to pass on responsibility for any manpower supply shortage to a higher agency - Districts to Regions, and Regions to the DHSS.

These three observations on the 1979-88 Regional strategic plans point towards a need to examine the issue of implementation versus stated intentions, the Region's and the District's role in manpower planning, and ways in which manpower requirements are generated and supply achieved. The former task, of exploring the implementation problem, was beyond the scope and timescale of the research project. It nevertheless remains an important area for study, particularly so in the climate of further Regional and District strategic plans (1985-1994), the movement to general management in the NHS, and the pursuit of a closer monitoring role by the DHSS and the Regions of District Health Authorities through the Annual Review Process, manpower targets and cash limits. Against this backcloth, what was the context surrounding manpower planning in the 1984 survey?

Under the present government's policies for the NHS, a system of manpower targets and a vacancy review procedure have been promulgated (HC(83)16 and HC(84)2) (see Chapter 3, Table 3.2). It was thus of interest to see how this had affected Health Authorities' approach to manpower. Respondents were also asked to indicate the support given to them in this area by the Regional Health Authority and to outline their own role in the manpower process.

All the Districts, in response to the manpower targets exercise, had introduced vacancy reviews and were actively seeking to control numbers. Many respondents commented that these practices generated high levels of dissatisfaction with management, lowered morale, and resulted in unnecessarily long delays in appointments being made. Also as no respondent in the interview survey had ever had a vacancy or case of need refused, it seems likely that either each post was needed, and thus delays in appointing could result in inadequate levels of care, or that each department had 'closed ranks' and made certain that unquestionable cases of need were put forward. Thus such procedures may largely have been functioning in a symbolic manner to make the District seem to be doing something.

Amongst the personnel officers and nurses, the general view was that since the introduction of manpower targets in 1983 they had overridden manpower planning either 'completely', or 'partly' (Table 7.2). Comments were voiced such as 'we are now back to the beginning again (with our plans), as targets allow only minimum staff increases'; it is a 'nuisance factor' or 'an additional factor to take into account'. But not all viewed it in this way. As two District Personnel Officers commented, the manpower targets exercise was

'crude but it stimulated consideration of manpower .... (But) it will lose its effect if it continues in its current form'.

Table 7.2: Manpower Management and Control (%)

	ALLIED HEALTH PROFESSIONALS		NURSING			PERSONNEL
	Physio- therapy	Occupational Therapy	DNS (Community)	DNS (Elderly)	CNO	
Have manpower targets over- ridden manpower planning?						
* completely or partly?	41	31	63	54	63	52
* not sure?	28	34	0	23	0	12
* not at all?	31	34	36	23	36	38
Is there a vacancy review system?						
* yes	66	53	58	43	58	69
Was there any advice, guidance or support from the RHA?						
* yes	21	13	50	14	50	69

Further, manpower targets

'deflate expectations, but they have not
overridden manpower planning. The need is to
justify anticipated staff requirements on an
objective and competitive basis'.

A Chief Nursing Officer remarked more sceptically,
that

'in some instances people are seeing the
manpower ceiling as the point to aim at, rather
than measuring manpower needs in a constantly
changing clinical environment'.

Finally, the difficulty in meeting manpower
targets and financial cash limits was frequently
mentioned, especially problematic as they are not
coterminous; being underspent on one's budget need
no longer mean the recruitment of an additional
staff member, the saving being used instead perhaps
to offset overspending in another's budget.

As for the allied health professionals (AHPs) a
similar proportion indicated that the manpower
targets exercise had 'partly' or 'not at all'
affected their manpower planning. Indeed, within
occupational therapy, as its establishment was often
not achieved, the manpower targets had little
impact: 'there are more occupational therapy jobs
available than qualified staff'. But negative
comments too abounded:

'the paramount interest is a headcount -
thus the level of service to patients is bound
to be reduced'; or, 'planning is difficult
without flexibility to increase staffing levels
if necessary'.

It is worth noting that as many as a quarter of the
respondents were 'not sure' of the effect of this
exercise, explicable perhaps by the lack of
involvement of AHPs in mainline management.

Turning to the second part of the circular's
requirement - a vacancy review system - most
respondents knew of its existence, at least at the
senior levels in the organisation (the District
Personnel Officers and Chief Nursing Officers).
Amongst the AHPs and the community nurses, a
frequent comment was that while a vacancy review
procedure existed it did not affect them, permission
to replace coming almost automatically, but with

some delay. The criteria outlined to justify replacement of a vacancy varied. Professional judgement was mentioned in a few instances - 'unacceptable consequences if the post is not filled', 'an adverse effect on patient care', and 'the post is essential to maintain standards of care'. In the majority, workload based criteria were noted: for example, 'the work cannot be done if the post is not filled; the reasons why the work cannot be shared; and the effect on overtime and on-call if the post remains vacant'; 'a need to replace exists and money is available'; 'the level of service required, existing workload and the projected increase in hospital discharge'; 'the work needs to be done and cannot be absorbed elsewhere with greater efficiency, and funding is there to pay for it'.

The responsibility for defining staffing demands and their deployment lay with the Unit Management Team, with the District Personnel Officer or Unit Administrator co-ordinating initiatives. One Unit Administrator stated, 'I see heads of departments or unit management groups, interview separate departmental heads to talk about their level of input into the proposed service, and what the manpower implications are for them'. However, although this suggests a team based approach to demand estimation and deployment, the reality was somewhat different.

There existed in many instances a lack of knowledge concerning the criteria upon which manpower decisions were made. For example, a Unit Administrator was not able to identify the reasoning behind decisions made by the heads of department; 'I don't think there are any objective criteria that we use to be honest'. The administrator continued that what he tried to do was to evaluate work tasks. 'Instead of saying "right, there are so many beds, therefore, this generates so many nurses," there is the question ... what are the nurses going to be actually doing'. However, when asked about how staffing requirements were formulated, far less knowledge was revealed: 'I don't know where the nurses get their figures from, I just accept the nurse figures that they tell me'. Indeed, other respondents in that District acknowledged that bed occupancy was used to determine nurse staff demands. In addition, understanding the basis of Regional decisions concerning manpower was not widely known. As a personnel officer stated, when discussing the manpower implications of new capital developments, 'you get a list of what is allocated under the revenue cost, and no-one knows how these figures are worked out. It's frightening in the sense that you set up the service on that figure as that is all you have'.

Thus at the level of Unit and District administration there existed extensive lack of knowledge about how staffing demands were being formulated. It was the departmental heads or Director of Nursing Services who were seen as being responsible for calculating staffing demands and for determining the deployment of labour. Depending on the personal approach of the departmental head and her dominance over the local power structure, other individuals play a more or less influential role. For example, a consultant's special interest will not surprisingly affect deployment and demand, and also whether or not he/she accepts as unchangeable traditional means of manpower planning. In addition, professional interests were found to have a determining influence over the decision making process. As one member of a Unit stated,

'when an appointment has spin offs on other departments, especially medical, then the medical team tend to make sure that everything is cast iron before agreeing. Each member of the team tends to have the interests of their profession as the top priority, and speaks only for them'.

A similar picture came across in the postal survey. The AHPs and DNSs said their role was to both formulate demand and ensure the achievement of supply. The DPOs and CNOs had in addition a general advisory and consultative role. The CNO was seen to provide manpower planning support to the DNS, and the DPO and DMO to the AHPs. As for guidance or assistance from Regional Manpower Planners (Table 7.2), only the DPOs and CNOs indicated that they received it to any degree, and then it tended to be in the form of guidelines (norms) or ratios, seen either as 'of limited value', as 'stimulating thought', or as 'useful pointers'.

Finally, pressure from a higher tier has proved in recent years to be increasingly crucial. Many initiatives had only been taken as such a response. As one DPO stated, when discussing operational plans,

121

'in this District traditionally the manpower plan has been non-existent. With the Region's new emphasis in its plan, and the Government's emphasis on manpower, it's quite obvious that we have to do something. So this is our first attempt for 15 years to build something in on manpower'.

As regards the management dimension of the manpower process, it is clear that it is starting to take precedence, given the tight economic climate and pursuit of efficiency. The dual processes of manpower targets, associated criteria over filling vacancies and cash limits establish a 'control' environment. This may discourage creative planning and the exploration of alternative forms of service delivery and manpower types and provision, particularly given the emphasis on efficiency apart from effectiveness (Long and Harrison, 1985) and the potential resistance of the health professionals. It thus becomes even more important to explore the implementation of the plans. Were staff with the desirable characteristics recruited, and in the requisite mixes? What influence, if any, was exerted on the production dimension?

MANPOWER PLANNING DIMENSION

How then did heads of department decide upon the required numbers of staff and their deployment? The answer proved complex. Looking at all the respondents together, while 90% stated that their 'professional judgement' was employed, it was not used on its own. It was used either together with guidance in the forms of staffing norms (67%) or together with a workload based approach (33%) — that is the numbers of staff required in relation to tasks to be done, dependency levels of patients, and so on. Table 7.3 shows the picture for each staff group. It is valuable to look at each manpower group separately in order to instance similarities and differences.

Medical Manpower

The process for exploring the need for a new consultant post is usually set in motion within the Cogwheel machinery. Occasionally individual consultants argue the case, although most DMOs reported that the initiating point is a department or a division. The main alternative is where the

Table 7.3: Estimating Staffing Requirements (%)

Type of Approach	Physicians*	Physio-therapy	Occupational Therapy	DNS (Community)	DNS (Elderly)	CNO	Personnel
Professional judgement on its own	17	21	12	23	7	0	0
Professional judgement and norms	0	24	31	57	21	0	19
Professional judgement and workload based, or norms and workload based	83	52	44	19	64	75	62
Intend to change the approach used in the future (% Yes)	**	21	28	62	43	33	69

* The figures for physicians are estimates, based on responses to open ended questions.
** Not Applicable

123

DMO acts as the catalyst. It is evident that there is considerable variation across hospital consultants about the merit of increasing their numbers - as requested in the DHSS response to the <u>Short Report</u> (House of Commons, 1981). Individuals or departments typically press for increases in their own areas, but it is not unknown for recommendations to be made to encourage growth in other specialisms as a priority.

There is a further possibility of a request originating from the Region. This might occur in the case of a Regional specialty where the service is spread over more than one District. As one DMO observed,

> 'a specialist sub-committee of the Regional Medical Committee would pass the request direct to the RHA and the District Health Authority would be asked for its observations'.

An even more infrequent happening is where funds are made available from some outside agency.

For the most part, however, requests for new consultant posts emanate from the District itself, and most typically from an individual or groups of individuals working within a particular division. The District Management Team (DMT) or Health Authority may itself take action where gaps in service provision seem to have arisen, or where complaints have been made about the lack of an appropriate service.

The identification of need for a new consultant post is the next step. The criteria employed vary considerably across Authorities. One respondent implied that the factors mentioned diverge significantly depending on how involved the physicians were in the wider health service planning process.

> 'New consultant posts may be sought either by a Cogwheel Division or by myself (the DMO). In the latter case, the need is determined by gaps in the service. In the former, the usual ploy is to quote College norms backed up by workload figures including throughout, waiting lists and comparison of staff numbers with other districts'.

The criteria which are identified as confirming 'need' congregate in the following areas:

- workload (deaths and discharges, new outpatients, waiting lists, bed occupancy);
- service needs, priorities, teaching/training requirements; inter-District/Region/National comparisons or physician-to-population ratios or College staffing norms; and
- changing medical practice (consequence of new capital schemes).

The overall impression is that the quality of data leaves much to be desired. Respondents pointed to the difficulties of obtaining valid and reliable 'quantifiable' information, which was directly related to demands for services in the locality.

> 'There is a need to support arguments with hard data ... but things are never as easy as they look, activity data and waiting lists never adequately reflect need. A case in point was the third cardiac surgeon appointed to relieve pressure; he created a new reservoir of demand'.

Nevertheless, there seemed to be a growing acceptance of a standardised checklist which would enable bids for consultant posts to be evaluated in terms of their revenue consequences, and in some cases, of their estimated benefit. In those Districts which have introduced such a procedure, the usual requirement is that consequential costs are estimated by appropriate medical and administrative personnel. One Authority has included the following for consideration in any application for a new consultant post:

- firstly, general objectives of the appointment;
- secondly, specific objectives (such as the likely effect on waiting lists, standard of treatment, and length of in-patient care, as well as medical productivity generally);
- thirdly, the effect of the appointment on diagnostic and support services, on other medical personnel, on nursing staff, on paramedical staff, on other staff; and
- non-staff resource implications.

The DMO respondents generally inclined to the view that physicians could not expect to have an application for a new post treated seriously unless due attention was given to the wider revenue consequences, although the amount of detailed information required varied enormously.

A further aspect in considering the implications of appointing a new consultant is highlighted by the mention made by DMOs of the importance of reaching agreement on a detailed job description. These will often be submitted to higher Authorities, as well as to the current consultant body. DMOs also mentioned the significance of achieving an agreed priority for the proposed new consultant posts, although non-physicians often charge medical committees with ignoring this issue. One Region has introduced a system to replace the annual bidding mechanisms which incorporate discussions across local consultants, the DMO and Regional Medical Officers. The new posts are listed in terms of local priority. Within these systems some claim to detect a 'hidden' rule that bids reflect what Districts feel that they can achieve, rather than what that actually need. There is an often uneasy merger between local and national priorities.

The approval of a new consultant post depends on successfully passing through a variety of examination points at all levels of the service. A typical process involves the following:

. support from other consultants in the area;
. agreement from the appropriate Cogwheel Division;
. agreement from the Medical Executive Committee;
. agreement from the DMT;
. agreement from the District General Manager/ Health Authority;
. approval by the Regional Manpower Committee/RHA; and
. approval by the Central Manpower Committee/DHSS.

Several respondents report on the relative difficulty of negotiating a way through the District level bodies - at least compared with the higher Authorities. The fact that there is no single pathway for approval of posts in hospitals, the community, and general practice is sometimes felt to inhibit 'the synchronisation and efficient planning of medical services' (Carruthers, 1984, p.286). For such critics of the existing system, a more co-ordinated approach to manpower planning is required within medicine, as well as other services.

One associated issue is the extent to which the initiation and approval of manpower bids amongst the medical community forms an integral part of the overall health planning system. A widely voiced criticism suggests that too much planning of medical services proceeds in isolation from the broader planning process and cycle with evident threats to service provision. DMOs in fact are split in their opinion as to the consistency of medical manpower planning with overall strategic and operational plans. The pressure is to move towards a climate in which new posts are only released on the recommendation of the DMT to meet essential service needs, and to try to balance developments 'in line with the Authority's plans and total resources'. One Authority which exemplies this pattern reports that all new medical staff posts are treated as an integral part of the planning process. The main steps followed entail:

1   issue of planning guidelines to the Divisions in early January;
2   dispatch of development proposals, including staffing bids to the Service Planning Department for analysis and collation; this is accompanied by a detailed outline of need encompassing a statement of objectives, expected output and outcome, quantified where possible, consequences for other services and an indication of how the proposal relates to the care group strategy;
3   staffing proposals are then considered by the Medical Executive Committee (MEC) and the DMT in relation to overall service needs;
4   the DMT then recommends a two year development programme for discussion and approval by the Health Authority in October; and
5   also in October, the District meets with the Region to indicate the posts for inclusion in the Region's medical manpower programme, and to request that manpower approvals be obtained where necessary. The whole thrust of such a system is 'to ensure that proposals and options are fully debated and that priorities are decided on the basis of service need'.

Most of the respondents indicated that the

procedures followed for establishing the need for and approval of new junior medical staff paralleled those outlined for new consultant positions. The obvious contrast stemmed from the quite different scope for creating new posts for juniors. The District guidelines that followed DHSS recommendations to increase the number of consultants and hold the number of junior medical staff varied markedly according to the survey. Several replied that the District Authority had no policy in this area, while others reported considerable opposition to establishing numerical parity between consultant and junior medical staff.

There was general agreement that it was difficult, if not impossible, to create new posts. However, there were several notable expections: for example, in Districts' developing new hospitals, or where the current proportion of junior doctors was low in national terms. For the most part, DMOs indicated that their Region had frozen any development of new posts, although some latitude for growth of particular grades was reported. The picture is complicated by DMOs in the same Region referring to contrary Regional directives.

In the main, Senior Registrar and Registrar posts are subject to especially stringent controls. If the RHA is informed of an available post, Districts are invited to bid. This entails detailed consideration through the various medical committees and management groups. Most obviously, the District has to assess how any such post fits into wider funding priorities.

The DHSS has been particularly keen to restrict Senior House Officer posts, and most DMOs indicated that a freeze on new posts in this grade had been demanded. Some respondents indicated that this applied to overall numbers, and that some redeployment within the Region was allowed. The consultants were generally extremely difficult to budge on this matter, and the criteria for identifying a need for juniors was reported to contain a strong 'random aspect', or to be based on 'historical precedent', or the power of individual consultants. In consequence, there were few illustrations of the successful transfer of a post between specialisms or Districts. The most likely opportunities for flexibility arose in very particular circumstances: closure of a unit, or services; meeting national training requirements; or ensuring adequate rota and off-duty arrangements.

Most flexibility or possibilities of new posts were concentrated in the pre-registration House Officer grades, and in the non-training grades, particularly Clinical Assistants. In the case of the former, a Regional target was usually fixed and appropriate specialty committees submitted proposals. These would have to be approved by the University on the educational content, before any application went to the RHA. Overall, it appears to be accepted that there will be little further increase in junior medical posts.

Nursing

Looking at the three groups of nursing respondents, again professional judgement together with either norms (in the community nursing context particularly, and the elderly to a much lesser extent), or workload based approaches was the standard. The workload approaches employed were the Telford Formula (46%), the Aberdeen Formula (23%), the Cheltenham Method (12%), the Goddard method (8%), and the Leicester, Oxfordshire and Rhys Hearn Care Package (4% each).

The use of two approaches was seen as valuable, to 'cross-check' views expressed. For example, the Telford Formula was used to compare against the Regional norm, or to supplement the sister's professional judgement (the formula builds on a systematic assessment of the ward sister's judgement). Where the Aberdeen Formula was used (predominantly in one RHA), professional judgement, it was pointed out, had to be employed to cover the '50% or so of areas not catered for (eg in mental illness)'. Further, it was remarked that there are 'no generally agreed (national) formula' (cf DHSS, 1984a), and thus 'the use of professional judgement is more acceptable locally'. The problem of 'the non-quantifiable aspects of nursing' was also referred to, often to justify use of professional judgement.

In two of the fifteen Districts explored in the interview survey, such workload based methods were being used with the aim of improving service provision. For example, in the District using the Cheltenham formula, nursing officers and sisters were encouraged to use the data from the dependency study criteria in order to evaluate and improve standards of care.

'We have had an impact on standards; as

129

recent data on workload showed, it closely correlated with staff because the nursing officer is now using our information and moving staff around, and looking at and anticipating the needs, recognising problems and matching resources'.

However, without exception, the methods or formulae adopted were perceived by respondents to have a more important usage, that is, to provide a scientific backing to the nurse's professional judgement. Thus,

'(the) system has been accepted by the Treasurer and once you go and say the dependency on ward X has increased, therefore we need Y number of nurses, they appear to accept it. At the minute it's difficult for us to go to them and say the workload on a ward has increased when all we can show them is higher patient turnover. We know that numbers of patients don't equal workload'.

Thus, although it is stated that formulae were being used to determine the demand for staff, whether they were adhered to on a day to day basis was questionable. They were often used for political expediency.

Notwithstanding a movement towards a more 'scientific' process for estimating nursing numbers and deployment, a predominance of what one DNS described as 'feeling what's right' still prevailed.

'I don't use those fancy formulas like Telford or Cheltenham or anything as I don't know anything about them; I use ... a sort of feel really, and experience. It's very difficult to teach anyone that. There is nothing scientific about it, you feel what's right'.

Thus, professional judgement was seen as a critical basis for the formulation of manpower demands at the District level. The DNS was dependent upon her nursing officers and sisters being able to feed back to her their own observations and knowledge of the ward situation. 'You use your own observations and what your nursing officers tell you'. The nursing officers and sisters would inform the DNS that, for example, babies were not getting fed on time, and therefore more staff were necessary. This view was reinforced by another DNS who stated that norms were

not really wanted for defining 'who' and 'how' many
staff were required as she expected her sisters to
be able to identify problems and to be responsible
for running the ward. The DNS must therefore know
her staff well; good staff to management
understanding is essential or else the ward will
not run smoothly. Such an approach has many
advantages. Because the DNS relies on her staff for
planning manpower, the system is very flexible and
day to day decisions about the deployment of staff
can be made quickly in response to ward
circumstances. Also the staff preferences for
working hours and conditions could be accommodated
easily which, as one DNS felt, increased the
efficiency of the ward and staff commitment.

The interviews thus revealed that staff at ward
level are largely making day to day planning
decisions, and are relied upon by nurse managers to
do so without the use of any scientific formula. For
example, as one DNS stated when asked what equalled
adequate staffing,

> 'the subjective dependency of the patients,
> because we haven't got any scientific method of
> dependency, we use the sister's professional
> judgement, she knows what her workloads are,
> the type of patient she's got, whether they
> were high dependency or low'.

But with the general belief that only processes
marked with a scientific stamp of approval are
valid, the important role that professional
judgement plays at ward level is often ignored or
perceived as invalid. Consequently, manpower
demands and deployment of staff are phrased in terms
of 'scientific' norms, statistics, and formulae, in
order to be acceptable to management and to protect
the profession's interests.

> 'Well you have to say that you are using this
> formula or that formula when reporting back to
> District - you have got to make it look good,
> it's all very well if I say to you I look at
> need or the population, but I don't'.

A veneer of objectivity is imposed on a
subjective process. At the same time, a Chief
Nursing Officer emphasised the need for consultation
and the importance of the sisters' judgement;

> 'in the hospital where we have got the highest

proportion of trained staff, they realise that they need the numbers, but not such a technical mix, and are now committed to reducing it and getting it right, which I don't think we would have achieved if we hadn't got a consultative method'.

In the community sector, the lack of workload based measures was frequently referenced. The resort to norms, however crude, were seen as 'giving a common baseline, and in any case, nothing else is available'. 'No adequate way to assess workload in the community' was noted. The future was seen by 63% to hold the need for developing an alternative, and particularly a workload based approach, especially so given that the norms are outdated (based on the Jameson Report). Several respondents indicated their intentions to 'assess each General Practice annually regarding workload, by patient type, diagnosis, dependency' and take into account the time spent on travel and with each patient.

As for advantages and disadvantages, the speed of the application of norms, and the positive strengths of professional judgement and the Telford approach in terms of consultativeness and adaptability to local needs were acknowledged. But, the 'lack of a scientific base' to professional judgement, the difficulties in trying to explain it to colleagues in other disciplines, and the 'subjective basis' of the Telford approach were also noted. On the community side, norms were seen as being 'too broadbrush, taking no account of local age distributions, social class, ethnic groups, etc', and more incisively as 'being not clearly defined as to what they relate to and how they were originally arrived at'. Changes in the future for all three groups of nurses were then unsurprisingly indicated to be the use of 'more objective/ scientific' approaches. In the elderly sector, use of the Rhys Hearn Care Package and the Cheltenham Method were noted. The CNOs also referred to the Cheltenham approach, Telford, the use of Regional guidelines and revised performance indicators, and GRASP.

The determination of the required skill mix also revealed similar processes, although any consideration of the overall mix of skills necessary for the provision of care, was token rather than perceived. One Unit Administrator stated,

'No we don't look at it globally, in fact I don't know anywhere that does. In my perception people in the NHS work in incredibly watertight compartments'.

The general approach to decisions taken at the departmental head level is to accept what has always been the mix in the past and old established norms. When change has been considered, it has, in most cases, been to increase the percentage of qualified to unqualified staff, and thus the degree of specialism. As a DNS stated,

'the care of the elderly has been seen as back-breaking work (with) little mental stimulation and that's what we have tried to change; we've tried to talk about improvements and approaches to care that have appeared to be more professionally oriented'.

Thus the base line criteria for determining the mix of skills is professional interests. In addition, professional approaches to care are advocated to encourage more qualified staff into a particular area.

Physiotherapy and Occupational Therapy

For both physiotherapy and occupational therapy, while norms existed, they tended to have little status. The norms were derived by the relevant professional body, based in occupational therapy on 'professional judgement of experienced staff'. Norms of the Association of District and Superintendent Chartered Physiotherapists (ADSCP), the British Association of Occupational Therapists (BAOT), the College of Occupational Therapists, and the British Geriatrics Society (BGS) were referred to. Some, notably those of the ADSCP, were highly specific according to the differing working locations of staff (geriatrics, orthopaedics). The 'lack of recognised norms' were referred to frequently. However such norms were criticised in several Districts as inflexible, providing no evaluation of workload, and lacking any degree of consultation with those at the local level.
    In this context, a combination of professional judgement and workload based approaches was employed: 'cases and non-patient contact, by grade of physiotherapist, plus an allowance for study leave, sickness, and annual leave'. But the 'lack

133

of involvement' of AHPs in the planning process, and a 'lack of awareness of the role of the occupational therapist' were frequently mentioned. Indeed, it was commented that 'an occupational therapy service was being built from nil, at the demand of other staff (nurses and consultants)'. Finally, professional judgement was often supported as it built on 'many years of experience', and was sensitive to patient needs and the local situation, 'getting the "feel" of the pressures on staff'.

In terms of advantages and disadvantages, the AHP respondents were as one in commenting on the lack of recognised norms and their disregard - 'the Health Authority is not inclined to aspire to the guidelines (of the BAOT)'. Such professional norms were in any case seen as 'minimum standards' and only of particular use in planning new developments. Professional judgement also was unacceptable, fallible and potentially biased. As one respondent remarked, it was 'seldom effective adopting professional management tactics'. More damningly, one commented that 'it is difficult to substantiate claims based on professional judgement; and even if one can, no-one is interested as there is no money'.

In terms of the future, neither the occupational therapists nor physiotherapists were intending to change their approach to estimating staffing requirements. For as many commented, they 'would like to look for alternative methods, but where from?'. In the context of the non-acceptance of professionally defined standards, their non-achievement (due in part to supply difficulties) and the apparent low priority given to these two groups' contribution to patient care, this negative attitude is unsurprising. Those who intended to change their approach pointed, like their nursing and personnel colleagues, to the use of workload based approaches, 'once basic staffing is achieved', planning on demographic data, for instance, related to clinical needs, or job evaluation. Performance indicators as a refinement to the professional norms were also noted.

Personnel Officers: The Co-ordinators

Amongst the so called co-ordinators of the manpower process - the personnel officers - two general opinions were voiced. Firstly, norms tempered by professional judgement, taking into account features of the local situation, was one general approach: 'a combination of methods is used; where norms exist and are proven, they are used; if the norms are not acceptable locally, then professional judgement is employed'. The other opinion was summed up in the phrase 'a general move from the subjective to the objective'. One respondent observed that

'the most scientific approach is work measurement; but there is professional resistance to it. The further one moves into A and C (administrative and clerical), P and T (professional and technical) and medical groups, the greater the reliance on professional judgement'.

In the context of AHPs, one DPO remarked that 'if you don't trust the norms, then professional judgement is bound to be used'.

Another major influence over the manner in which the demand for staff is evaluated is that of crisis intervention. In general, the requirement for additional staff was argued for on the basis that either staff or the service had reached a breakdown point. For example, 'the Chief Occupational Therapist comes and says she just can't cope, so then you get a new occupational therapist'. Of course the bid for such staff will not be put to the District in such terms; instead, criteria such as norms will be employed. However, the initial identification of a need for more staff is dependent on a key individual intervening at a crisis point, with little analysis of future needs. Thus as a DPO argued,

'yes, we are very bad in the NHS at identifying future problems and acting upon them; we, for example, don't take up the issue of a key individual retiring in a few years and train someone up. I am afraid that I don't know of anywhere that's done'.

The advantages and disadvantages of the current approaches were pointed out by the respondents. Workload approaches were seen as most easy to justify, and carrying greatest weight, followed by norms (on relationships, roles and numbers) which were seen as providing consistency over time, and as being really the only option to identify earlier on the staffing requirements for professions with a long training lead time. On the other hand, norms were seen as problematic as they were often out of date ('when were they last revised?') and perhaps of little relevance to a local situation, and sometimes because they tended to be viewed as 'tablets of stone'. Professional judgement too was seen as 'often overgenerous'. Finally, while workload approaches were seen as 'best', a lack of resources to adopt this approach was noted.

As for the future, 69% of the DPOs indicated that they intended to change the approach used to estimate demand. A move to a 'more scientific approach', towards using 'activity/workload based measures', notably with a link to 'more refined performance indicators', was the intended modification. As one respondent commented, 'there is always room for modification, by improved judgement, norms, and modern technology and methods'.

A Multi-Disciplinary Team Approach

Respondents were asked to comment on the general manpower planning approach adopted in their District. Nearly all respondents (95%) indicated that staffing requirements were estimated on a staff group basis, 'at least to some extent' (Table 7.4). The common view was that 'yes, it is the way line managers assess their own needs'; in an 'uniprofessional approach'; 'historically, this is the case'; 'separately managed and funded staff groups'. 'Little interdisciplinary dialogue' was noted, and 'little co-ordination between disciplines'. More directly,

'every staff group is defensive; this has been intensified by recent manpower cuts; there is no agreed approach to a multi-disciplinary approach'.

Such a remark was echoed by another:

'demand is assessed by care group (for example, the elderly, children) and analysed by staff group; the current emphasis on "direct" and "indirect" patient care (under the manpower targets, circular HC(84)2) hampers across discipline concern'.

And again,

Table 7.4: Manpower Planning as a Multi-Disciplinary Approach (%, all groups)

	Totally	To Some Extent	Not At All/ Unacceptable Option	Don't Know
Estimating staffing requirements on a staff group basis	74	21	4	1
Planning staffing requirements across staff groups: a multi-disciplinary approach	8*	80**	4	8
Pursuit of the WHO objective of manpower planning, 'specifying teams and their composition'	0	46	51	3

NOTES

* currently in use
** either seen as a useful approach and beginning to be adopted, or seen as a useful approach and pursuing it in the future

137

'medical manpower planning is out of the
control of the District - the cost of the
consultant's tail. Even now rather than lose a
consultant post it is accepted without
assessing or providing for the full revenue
cost'.

Further, when one respondent who was responsible
for medical manpower was asked how, when an area
for service development has been identified, the
medical manpower requirements were determined, the
answer was illuminating.

'Look, it doesn't work like that, you start by
appointing a consultant and then according to
his interests the number of other staff are
determined, and the appropriate service is
developed'.

The AHPs emphasised their relative isolation,
observing that 'nurses and doctors have direct
representation on the DMT and UMT, and also more
norms are available'. '(We have to) strive
independently for any staff increase. I am asked
for staff bids without knowing what other
professions' demands for staff are'. Further, 'a
shortfall of occupational therapists means that
their true worth and potential is never estimated,
except in geriatrics'. No co-ordinated approach
occurs. 'Professions are very protective of their
own disciplines and fail to appreciate the need for
an overview'. 'Each group has its own conception of
its contribution to care; the total of all is never
looked at'. 'Each discipline has to "fight for
itself"'. 'I was never invited to discuss staffing
demands in conjunction with other professions'.
It is hardly surprising then to see the
picture presented in Table 7.4 regarding the
alternative of a multi-disciplinary team based
approach to manpower planning. As for the WHO
objective of manpower planning (as being 'to specify
the number of teams and the composition needed to
improve the level of health up to a proposed level'
- Mejia, 1978) 'planning by care group' was seen as
potentially leading to such a methodology, with
provisos regarding the 'historical situation'
('those who have staff/posts keep them; those who do
not do without', and 'planning revolves around beds
not manpower') and difficulties in defining 'health'
and 'service objectives', and in orientating
services towards the community, prevention and

rehabilitation. 'A lack of co-operation between <u>all</u> disciplines at times, and often between the NHS and Social Services' was noted, as too was 'poor inter-departmental communication, especially in the teaching hospital'.

'Specifying teams and their composition' was thus not seen by the majority as being a description of their current activity. Rather

> 'the team care approach has yet to be developed in the NHS. Priority is given to treating ill health rather than planning a level of health for the community it serves'.

On a more positive note,

> 'no - it is disjointed; I am sure if this (approach) did take place in a more organised fashion, better patient care would result'.

Notwithstanding these negative comments, the potential of a multi-disciplinary approach was recognised. Indeed, it was perceived as 'useful' by about 88% of respondents. A small proportion was pursuing it in specific areas, and more were starting to. Its potential in areas of mental illness, mental handicap and geriatrics (including community liaison) was pointed out. 'Understanding the role and contribution of other staff to patient care would be a good idea'. Limitations and difficulties were also recognised.

> 'Yes - this approach is useful; but there is a discrepancy with medical manpower planning. New consultant appointments can still occur without a satisfactory assessment of other staffing requirements needed to support them'.

Further, 'there are too many inter-disciplinary disputes to be resolved before we can move in that direction'. In the community area, such an approach was seen to be essential given the developing specialisation there 'in order to avoid unnecessary overlap'. In a more administrative vein, a personnel officer argued that the approach was useful because of the 'interdependence of functions. The manpower planner has to obtain a corporate view, leading to a balance between functions, within financial parameters'. 'This is what is required to get the best level of expertise', commented a physiotherapist; but, 'personalities and professional insecurity make it very difficult'. It too can assist where 'difficulties in recruiting one professional occur', and where 'there is no strong professional divisions' (eg in psychogeriatrics).

Finally, the organisational isolation of occupational therapy was expressed: 'priorities are dominated by administration, medics and nursing'; and 'I approve (of the approach) - I sent my ten year strategic plan to about sixty colleagues; I did not receive any others in return'. Entrenched attitudes, professional rivalry, suspicion, and attention on 'what the service costs, not is it essential and/or effective' seem to stand in the way. In sum, an integrated approach '... is not operated at present; if it was it would give a better balance to patient needs'.

The above discussion relating to the planning dimension of the manpower process has focussed on the way staffing numbers were generated. Several observations can be made. Firstly, a general movement towards the adoption of some form of workload based approach is occurring, across all manpower groups. While professional judgement still plays a dominant role, it is not perceived as sufficient; evidence of implications on workload and services to patients is required in addition. Reference back to the pressures noted within the management dimension may point to the underlying reason for this. Notwithstanding its cause, this process was evident among physicians (in the context of arguing for the creation of new posts), nurses (to justify the filling of any post falling vacant due to staff turnover), and allied health professionals (whose position is in any case a little problematic given the sometimes limited recognition of their role). The potential impact of claims in the interest of professional status and clinical autonomy should not be forgotten. Secondly, norms whilst still seen as valuable in outline planning are not surprisingly being downgraded in importance as providing a firm indication of staffing levels. Significantly, the views of the current manpower co-ordinators (personnel) express a desire for a more 'scientific' approach, acitivity and workload based. Finally the planning of manpower requirements is carried out predominantly on a staff group by staff group basis. A multi-disciplinary team approach has been adopted in only a few areas, namely amongst services for the elderly and the mentally ill. The relevance of professionalism must be noted. Indeed, it is easier to plan manpower by staff group given current professional interest groups and their relative power positions in the organisation. One is left with the impression that manpower is planned more to support professional interests than to provide manpower teams with skills and experiences appropriate to meet patient needs.

MANPOWER PRODUCTION: ATTEMPTS TO MATCH DEMANDS

Once manpower requirements have been formulated, the next question is how to set about ensuring that manpower with the desirable qualifications, skills and experience is produced and recruited in line with the plans. How were Districts in the survey actually approaching this issue? An uniformity in approach was apparent, even in Districts which had traditionally possessed very different manpower supply problems. Responses to difficulties in supply covered a limited range, not least because many facets of supply were assumed to be outside the sphere of influence of the organisation.

In the interview survey, answers to questions concerning manpower supply tended to be vague, revealing a lack of consensus. For example, one member of a Regional manpower planning team stated,

> 'there are certainly a lot of problems in recruitment in specific areas, such as occupational therapists, as this Region is particularly poor in its training schools; in fact, I don't know if we have got one. We have, I think, got a Physiotherapist School'.

Regions also tended to respond to supply problems by perceiving them as a District responsibility. Furthermore, any in-depth analysis of supply was precluded by the concentration of manpower controls, targets and cash limits, again suggesting the increasing dominance of the management dimension.

At the District level, not surprisingly more attention was given to supply issues in areas with traditional recruitment problems. However, consideration of turnover rates and the need or desirability of retraining staff was largely ignored. In response to questions about recruitment problems, several solutions were offered. One major response was that an advertising campaign would have been mounted which consisted largely of changing the manner in which a post was advertised, such as improved format or wider publicity. These campaigns were designed to attract both newly qualified and unemployed staff. This for most Districts was the first option.

Substitution and role enlargement was another policy considered, although it aroused strong professional objections. Substitution was recognised as a relatively common practice within a profession, although not across professions, even where tasks would appear to lend themselves to such an approach. It was often seen as the only way of maintaining the service in situations of low recruitment. For example, juniors often 'act up' for seniors. In the midwifery service, the DMS regularly employed staff nurses to cover the special care baby unit where recruitment of midwives was difficult; qualified midwives in the circumstances were not thought necessary.

The reason offered was not that the tasks were too specialised.

> 'The problem is of professionalism. Nurses won't cut toe nails, and the foot care department won't let them. The old community ones would do it, but the new ones don't see that as their job, ... and you can't get round this'.

Professional groups are anxious to protect their authority, and thus oppose any move which could reduce their control. In addition, manpower targets have inhibited such initiatives. Managers have been forced to be very aware of the role and function of all their staff, and rather than advocate substitution, departmental heads have condemned it. For if a nurse is allowed to extend her role into physiotherapy, then fewer physiotherapists will be needed. Alternatively, as a CNO remarked;

> 'I wouldn't necessarily condone an extension of the nurse's role, especially with manpower targets which have made people more aware of the staff they have got, and the use they should be making of them .... If we have got so many staff that we can let them do occupational therapy, physiotherapy, or act as

escorts, then we have got too many staff'.

Similarly, training was felt to be entirely within the sphere of each professional group. Little consideration was given to the training of staff with specific skills in order to match future needs and service developments, as no-one at the District managerial level had any real input into the content of basic training courses. Although Districts did provide some evaluation of the numbers of entrants into training schools, this input tended to be short term and fairly crude, and consisted of raising issues such as, 'will there be enough, or too many, qualified nurses in three years time to supply our needs?' Longer term implications of say the drop in available 18 year olds by 1990, or changes in the role of the nurse, were not considered. Thus the input into training tended to consist of short-term responses to immediate fluctuations in the demand for staff.

In general, the concept of putting resources into retraining qualified staff or responding to shortages by considering the needs of the predominately female work force were also not raised For example, while increased flexibility of working hours was not uncommon, it was not considered to be an entirely adequate solution; the recruitment of of full-time staff was the first priority. Senior management frequently expressed prejudiced attitudes against part-time staff. For example, a Unit Administrator stated,

'you find that you are taking people only on their terms and not meeting the service needs, so that's the problem; and also you don't get the commitment either, they just don't get involved in the job or what's going on'.

However, most departmental heads advocated flexible working hours as one solution to supply problems. For example, while, as a DNS argued, one drawback of part-time workers is a lack of continuity of care,

'part-time staff are extremely valuable, we couldn't function without them. My night staff are entirely part-timers, in fact I employ largely part-timers and they work exceptionally hard'.

In terms of attracting staff to a District or specialism where there was a shortage, more flexible working hours were offered as an incentive, especially within the nursing profession.

Nursing and the medical profession had both adopted practical measures to attract women back into the service after a child rearing break. Numerous Districts had employed 'back to nursing campaigns' and retraining schemes including a 'woman doctor' retainer scheme. However, attitudes to a staff creche were far less positive. Senior mangement tended to reject them as posing too many 'managerial hassles' and as wasteful of resources, although in the vast majority of Districts, the flexibility of providing a creche or similar facilities had apparently not been investigated. The contention was that demand was low. As a DNS stated,

> 'I can't remember a nurse ever coming along and saying "have you got creche facilities"; they usually say, "I have made arrangements, what job have you got to offer?"'

However, this ignores two important issues: firstly, that a woman who was seen as not having made adequate child-care arrangements would be unlikely to be given employment; and secondly, the 'pool' of women who would return, but who are unable to find child-care provisions, and who therefore do not apply.

Although some initiatives were taken to attract staff into a District or particular specialties with supply problems, retraining qualified and experienced staff was scarcely considered. The area of discriminatory practices was not an issue, and thus female labour resources were not being developed as effectively as possible. For some in senior management the preponderance of women in the NHS workforce was a 'manpower problem'. A Regional officer stated, 'this service is 99% women, and in all truth, if we could get more men in we would have far less manpower problems and wouldn't be in such a mess'(!)

Broader consideration of supply issues is also inhibited by the manner in which manpower issues come onto the policy agenda. Firstly, an issue is seen as requiring action only once it has reached a crisis point; thus high turnover rates are not an issue as long as staff can be replaced. Secondly, manpower planning is seemingly determined by the interests of conflicting professional groupings, rather than by a patient centred outlook. Thus staff shortages can be responded to by 'poaching staff' from other hospitals, units or Districts, as professional or area interests are more paramount than looking at the needs of the whole national organisation. As one DPO stated, 'the health service as you probably realise runs by taking people from other hospitals'.

The general responses to supply problems as uncovered in the interview survey were very restricted in their range; and where they failed, little remained. When asked 'what happens to the service when appointments are not made?' the majority indicated that the service would not be provided or standards would decline. For example, a nurse planner stated that

'the service would just not develop. We have this problem with a Consultant Psychiatrist and until the appointment the service just stood still'.

This situation was the same in the community where it was stated that, 'they would have to cope', and coping meant 'no new referrals, closure of sessions, or that people are seen but less often as in chiropody'. This suggests that service provisions may have actually deteriorated because isues of production have not been addressed or raised.

Building on the above findings from the interview survey, in the postal questionnaire respondents were asked whether they had ever experienced any problems recruiting staff. Table 7.5 summarises the responses. All groups had experienced difficulties occasionally, while the community nurses and occupational therapists especially had frequent problems. Indeed, occupational therapy stands out as having difficulties 'most of the time' (56%), echoed in comments on the questionnaires of a 23%, or a 43% shortage in supply.

As to which groups were found most difficult to recruit, the AHPs were most often mentioned. Within these, the occupational therapists reported problems in recruiting all grades (66%), while amongst the physiotherapists it was evenly split between Basic and Senior/Superintendent. In nursing, the community nurses experienced considerable difficulties with health visitors (67%) and district nurses (52%), while the DNS for the Elderly spoke of staff nurses. Finally, the CNO respondents highlighted the recruitment of registered mental nurses (50%) and

A Survey of Manpower Practices

Table 7.5: Problems in Recruiting Staff (%)

Staff Group	Never	Occasionally	Frequently or most of the time
Physiotherapy	10	62	27
Occupational Therapy	0	22	78
DNS (Community)	4	48	48
DNS (Elderly)	21	50	29
CNO	12	46	42
Personnel	6	63	31

specialist nurses such as theatre nurses and midwives (33%), as well as community nurses (17%).

Against this backcloth of moderate (for most groups) and extensive difficulties (for occupational therapy and community nursing) in recruiting particular grades of staff, respondents were also asked about the strategies they had used or were using to try to overcome such problems. Table 7.6 shows the responses for the fourteen strategies listed on the questionnaire. The most used were an advertising campaign, a register or bank of ex-employees willing to take on work, increasing the amount of part-time openings and changing the staffing mix. Such comments apply across all the staff groups.

As to the success of such strategies, most groups were optimistic. In contrast, 66% of the occupational therapists indicated that the strategies had not worked. Which ones were actually seen as most successful varied from group to group. The DPOs with their more general co-ordinating role and their more corporate perspective identified the advertising campaign as most potent (69%), followed by a register or bank of ex-employees (25%), and 'back to nursing' campaigns or expanding a training school. Amongst the nurses, there was less agreement; all mentioned part-time openings as a key item. Others of note were 'back to nursing' campaigns, expanding or opening a training school, and changing the staff mix. For the AHPs the advertising campaign was seen as important (25%), upgrading posts (physiotherapy 31%), increasing part-time openings (21%), and 'other' strategies. Amongst this 'other' category, occupational therapists mentioned 'the need to establish a reputation for the service' 'to sell the profession', 'to build up its image', and the rotation of posts (also noted frequently by the physiotherapists), or attracting students on placement to areas of staffing difficulty with the hope that they will then choose to go back to those areas upon completing their training.

The above exploration of Districts' approaches to the area of manpower production has shown their limited attempts to influence the educational and training sector, either in terms of basic, post-basic or continuing education. Refresher courses are available only to a certain extent and only to meet local and periodic manpower recruitment difficulties. Strategies most commonly employed to meet manpower requirements tended to focus on

Table 7.6: Stategies Used to Overcome Difficulties in Supply (%)

	Physio-therapy	Occupational Therapy	DNS (Community)	DNS (Elderly)	CNO	Personnel
1 Advertising campaign	59*	78*	60	64	71	88*
2 'Back to nursing' campaign	11	25	15	36	58	75
3 Register/bank	44	56	70	79	92	81*
4 Labour survey	19	25	5	14	13	25
5 Attract more to take up training places	22	53	65*	14	39	31
6 Expand/open training school	11	38	20	0	52	44
7 Upgrade post	44*	50	10	50	13	44
8 Offer higher salary point	0	13	0	0	4	63
9 Increase part-time openings	56	78	85*	79*	74	69
10 Provide creche	19	31	25	21	39	50
11 Enlarge role	48	38	35	36	44	38
12 Change staff mix	56	63	55	86*	91	75
13 Retrain existing staff	59		25	29	44	38
14 Other**	41*	31*	20	0	22	31

* Strategy noted as the most successful by at least 25% of that group.
** See text for examples.

148

influencing those currently not in the NHS labour force to return to it, in itself a sensible ambition given the investment previously made in their training and education. However whether the educational institutions were producing persons with the relevant qualifications and skills was not addressed. This is perhaps not surprising given the lack of attention to the issue of roles in formulating manpower requirements, and the separation of the education sector, at least for doctors and allied health professionals from DHAs in the NHS. In addition, Districts appeared to be acting as separate bodies in terms of their recruitment and training policies, all competing for the same workforce, sometimes even between units within one District. It should also be noted that there is increasing competition between the NHS and the private sector over qualified manpower, a factor not explored in the study, as well as competition over payscales between the NHS and industry for its less qualified staff, and between the NHS and local authorities and general medical practitioners in the fields of chiropody and nursing respectively. Finally, while substitution and role enlargement were being discussed as a means of overcoming difficulties in recruitment, they tended to meet considerable professional resistance, with consequent effects on the scope and quality of the service provided to patients.

CONCLUSION

The interview and postal questionnaire survey of manpower practices within DHAs in England and Wales in 1984 suggests that Health Authorities which are different geographically and demographically, have responded to manpower issues and problems in strikingly similar ways, even where their manpower demand and supply were very different.

Several trends can be observed. Firstly, there was a general shift from the use of professional judgement and norms in estimating staffing requirements to the use of workload and activity based methods. This was summed up in the phrase of a 'movement from the subjective to the objective and scientific'. Secondly, manpower was planned by staff group. Indeed, strong professional resistance to multi-disciplinary co-operation was indicated. A minority saw this alternative approach as valuable; the specifications of manpower teams, their composition, and their link to changes in health were identified as the way forward for manpower planning. Thirdly, difficulties were often experienced in meeting manpower requirements, although these were generally overcome through the pursuit of multifarious supply strategies. However, chronic problems of labour shortage were noted for the occupational therapists. Fourthly, government policies on manpower targets were viewed ambivalently, but had reinforced a shift to justify vacancies on workload based criteria. Finally, the role of most of the respondents in manpower planning was to explore manpower requirements and pursue the achievement of their supply.

In addition, although on the surface clearly defined procedures and roles for the relevant individuals existed - for the calculation of manpower demands and for the exploration of supply - the manpower dimensions are characterised by numerous processes which are far from 'ordered' or put into a coherent framework. A District may define its role as centrally co-ordinating unit initiatives in manpower planning, and a Region as one of co-ordinating District initiatives and formulating longer term strategic plans. But these definitions ignore a host of influential groups and institutional political processes which determine the direction of the manpower process.

In summary, there is a lack of co-ordination and of integrating mechanisms between the three dimensions of the manpower process. Manpower requirements, in the planning phase, are formulated in terms of workload based approaches, in itself an interesting development with implications for deployment and skill mix (the management dimension). But the fundamental question of role definition - who does what, for whom, and why? - is not often raised; rather planning numbers remains within accepted role demarcations. Indeed, attempts at role enlargement and substitution meet professional resistance. Furthermore, little influence is exerted upon the production dimension, in terms of educational and training requirements. The survey data corroborates the lack of integration with the general planning process. As one administrator bemoans, progress is slow in '... preventing medical services from being planned in a vacuum and often unrelated to the health service needs of the community' (Carruthers, 1984, p. 286). The survey indicates the wider applicability of this observation. The lack of a team approach to planning manpower; little or no attempt to influence the educational and training sector, indeed its almost being left to another level or person in the organisation; professional self-interest, occupational control, and preservation of status: all these factors combine to act against an integration of the planning, production and management dimensions within the manpower process. There remains a large gap between theory and practice, to the detriment of the provision of staff with appropriate skills and experience to deliver the required service to meet patients' needs.

Chapter 8

PRIMARY HEALTH CARE - ASPECTS OF THE BRITISH
EXPERIENCE

WHO defines primary health care (PHC) in the
following manner as:

> '... meeting the basic health needs of each
> community through services provided as close
> as possible to where people live and work,
> readily accessible and acceptable to all,
> and based on full community participation'
> (WHO, 1985b, p.5-6).

Even amongst the exponents of PHC there is
disagreement about its most appropriate definition
and component parts. There is a further debate
about the gap between theory and practice.

In the British NHS, the predominant mode has
been to follow the distinction between hospital and
other services and to regard PHC as the concern of
the non-hospital sector. The latter provides the
first point of contact for patients with the health
service. It comprises those

> 'services that are provided by general
> practitioners, nurses, health visitors and
> other staff in the doctors' surgeries, in
> clinics, in special institutions for the
> handicapped and impaired and in the patients'
> home' (Hicks, 1976, p.1).

While this categorisation is indicative of the
mainstream approach in Britain, as a definition it
begs a number of crucial questions. There is an
immediate narrowing of the 'health' field by its
focus on institutional arrangements contained within
the NHS (for example, education, housing and social
services are effectively excluded), and by the
tendency to translate 'health care' into 'medical
care'. This also implies a view of health which is
overly concerned with treatment rather than

prevention or promotion - an impression conveyed in the charge that the National Health Service is more properly called a 'sickness service'.

As PHC has been re-interpreted to suit existing health service arrangements and philosophies, so it has been used to stimulate service innovations and developments. Aspects which have received support in Britain include the development of health care in the community, multi-disciplinary teams, health centres and changing roles for health care professions. The impact of PHC on the manpower process is also highly significant, as indeed the reception of PHC will be influenced by its manpower implications.

The aim of this chapter is to situate PHC in its British context. This is accomplished through a review of the organisational context and the particular division of responsibilities which places the onus for primary care on family practitioner and community services. The discussion then turns to current developments in PHC and implications for the future.

ORGANISATIONAL CONTEXT

The responsibility for PHC is divided between two statutory bodies: the District Health Authority (DHA) - formerly the Area Health Authority (AHA) - and the Family Practitioner Committee (FPC). Each has distinct duties or obligations to discharge which, although separate in a structural sense, are seen as providing the range of PHC services considered appropriate and necessary. FPCs were introduced in the wake of the reorganisation of the NHS in 1974. Each AHA was required to establish a FPC. But it was not a committee of the AHA in the conventional sense, at least in England and Wales. The reality was that FPCs were quasi-autonomous bodies, part of the structure of the AHA, but not really accountable to it. Most significantly, the FPC was largely outside the financial control of the AHA because it administered an 'open ended' budget which was directly allocated by the DHSS.

One of the many reasons for integrating the health structure in 1974 was to bring FPCs into the mainstream of the health services, and to involve them in wider health service planning. There were four major areas in which a close working relationship between AHAs and FPCs was considered advantageous. These can be briefly outlined as:

. to ensure that the views of the FPC, particularly as regards service planning, manpower development and attachment schemes, are made known to the AHA and its officers;

. to, in turn, keep the FPC informed of AHA plans, especially those which carry implications for the family practitioner services (FPS);

. to advise the FPC on any problems arising from its relationship with its independent contractors; and

. to provide general administrative and management advice to the FPC and its constituent sub-committees.

The AHA was responsible for all hospital and hospital-related services including so-called 'community services'. The latter covered such fields as community midwifery, district nursing, health visiting, chiropody, physiotherapy and community medicine. For its part, each FPC has had responsibility for four family practitioner services: general medical, general dental, opthalmic, and pharmaceutical. Through its officers the FPC administers the contracts and terms of service for the individual practitioners within these four general service areas. It also liaises with the Medical Practices Committee (MPC) concerning medical manpower, vacancies for GPs and future service developments. Together these family practitioner services and the community services administered by the AHAs have constituted what is generally referred to as PHC.

With effect from 1 April 1985, FPCs ceased to be dependent upon Health Authorities for staff and administrative arrangements and became independent public bodies, directly accountable for their activities to the Secretary of State for Health and Personal Social Services. One rationale for this change in status was to promote 'a closer working partnership to serve the interests of the community, especially in respect of primary health care' (DHSS, 1984b). It was envisaged that collaboration between FPCs and Health Authorities could be consolidated and fostered in two ways: an exchange of appropriate information; and commitment to health services planning.

The change in the organisational and

operational arrangements of FPCs is on the one hand largely symbolic in the sense that there will be little or no alteration in the manner in which the FPC administers the services under its jurisdiction. On the other hand, however, the change is of significance because it severs the links, which existed since 1974, between FPCs and local Health Authorities. The 1974 reorganisation was promoted as in the interests of integration and co-ordination. The 1985 changes could be seen, in this context, as a step backward to the situation pertaining before 1974 when the distinction between the different bodies responsible for health care was emphasised to such an extent that fragmentation and duplication of services occurred (DHSS, 1972). While the DHSS (1984b) is sanguine that the change will produce positive benefits, others are not optimistic that this will be so unless certain conditions are satisfied (Green and Rathwell, 1985).

Prior to the introduction of the legislation necessary for granting FPCs their independence the DHSS established a working group to consider ways in which collaboration between FPCs and DHAs could be encouraged (DHSS, 1984b). The working group argued that collaboration between DHAs and FPCs was only possible if the following precepts were accepted by both parties:

. a mutual understanding and respect for each other's role and responsibilities;

. the identification of areas of common interest and concern and the establishment and pursuit of common goals, policies and programmes in these areas;

. agreements concerning the sharing of information; and

. the creation of formal arrangements and informal links to secure co-operation between organisations by the simplest means and at levels appropriate to the functions concerned (p.5).

Health services planning was considered the common denominator for the translation of these precepts from ideal to reality. A number of informed commentators have warmly welcomed these changes, heralding them as a new era in the planning of primary care services (Pledger, 1984; Pursur, 1984; Wilcox, 1984). More cautious observers have suggested that such optimism is misplaced in that this organisational change for FPCs is not capable of producing a re-alignment of primary care services because it does not address (nor was it intended to) the fundamental issue of the manner in which the providers of primary care understand and discharge their responsibilities (Green and Rathwell, 1985).

The greatest impediment to effective collaboration, as the working party acknowledged, is the 'fact that hospital and community health services and family practitioner services are provided and administered in different ways' (DHSS, 1984b, p.6). This distinction is important. DHAs plan on the basis of local needs, national guidelines and policies, and within known financial resources and manpower constraints, whereas the activities of FPCs are defined by what individual practitioners decide to provide and how they elect to manage their services, but are not subject to the same financial limitations because of the fee-for-service principle. In consequence, changes in family practitioner services cannot be obtained in the same way as with the managed services of DHAs. The fact of the matter is that FPCs cannot speak for their constituents. Thus, in planning terms they are at a distinct disadvantage vis-a-vis Health Authorities. It is imperative that FPCs and DHAs find a meaningful way to plan together. This could be accomplished by each party jointly considering which goals should mould the planning agenda; the factors likely to constrain or enhance the implementation of agreed plans; and what the components should be for an efficient and effective primary health care service.

Achieving such an organisational change will not be easy given the different roles and responsibilities of the major actors in providing primary health care. The way the two bodies are funded is a major factor in structuring their individual concepts of primary health care and how they choose to apply them. In general, the artificial distinction between the family practitioner services (family doctors, dentists, opticians and pharmacists), the community health services (district nurses, community midwives, health visitors, community psychiatric nurses), and health related services (education, housing and social services) is likely to be maintained even though they are taken as constituting primary health care. If the joint planning efforts of FPCs and DHAs for primary health care services are to have any lasting impact, a quantum leap in conceptual terms is required necessitating a move away from a purely service devised notion of primary care to one constructed around a holistic view.

The discussion this far has outlined the organisational context in which PHC has developed in the NHS. Organisational structures and processes, as described for the situation in England and Wales, provide central parameters for the development of manpower policies for PHC. The health manpower process will now be examined in two of the principal FPS groups: firstly, general medical practitioners (GPs); and secondly, general dental practitioners (GDPs).

GENERAL MEDICAL PRACTITIONERS

According to Chaplin (1982) 'the general practitioner as family doctor is what makes the NHS unique among health care systems' (p.37), because the GP-patient relationship is a continuous one and not episode specific as with hospital treatment. This characteristic of continuing care is open-ended in the sense that patients are free to choose their GP, provided that the GP of their choice is willing to accept them. The Royal College of General Practitioners (RCGP) defined the GP as

> 'a licensed medical graduate, who gives personal, primary and continuing care to individuals, families and a practice population, irrespective of age, sex and illness' (quoted in Royal Commission Report, 1979, para. 7.17).

The goal is for the GP to accomplish this through the integration of physical, social and psychological factors and in conjunction with other primary health care team members. The delivery of PHC therefore necessarily extends beyond the experience of any single (medical) practitioner. The increasingly fluid perception of health care needs is a major reason for developing the team approach, at least insofar as it is believed that the physiological aspects of illness are increasingly difficult to separate from their social, environmental, cultural and psychosomatic origins (Noack, 1980).

Research into general practice offers a less

optimistic picture of the development of primary health care (Harding, 1981; Metcalfe, 1982; LHPC, 1981; Jefferys and Sachs, 1983). The Royal College of General Practitioners, in its evidence to the Royal Commission on the NHS, accepted that,

> 'our picture of the assets of good general practice must be balanced by the frank recognition that care by some doctors is mediocre, and by a minority is of an unacceptably low standard' (Report, 1979, para.7.28).

Others have suggested that the way so many GPs discharge their responsibilities falls between paternalism and human plumbing (McCormick, 1979).

There has, notwithstanding such criticism, been considerable change in the organisation and delivery of general medical services since the creation of the NHS, and especially in the last two decades. For example, there has been a significant growth in professional contact between GPs and non-medical health care practitioners. A survey of nurses in England and Wales working in the community in 1980 found that the vast majority regarded themselves as 'members of a primary health care team' and they rated their 'contacts and liaison with doctors' as good or very good. The close co-operation of health visitors and district nurses with family doctors is extending to encompass other community nurses (Dunnell and Dobbs, 1982, ch.5). Such claims imply that there has been a movement towards implementation of proposals in the Harding Report which argued forcefully in favour of primary health care teams. It is interesting to note its definition of the primary health care team:

> 'an interdependent group of general medical practitioners and secretaries and/or receptionists, health visitors, district nurses and midwives who share a common purpose and responsibility, each member clearly understanding his or her own function and those of the other members, so that they all pool skills and knowledge to provide an effective primary health care service' (p.2).

Despite these claims that the team approach to primary health care has become more popular with both doctors and nursing staff, it is perhaps surprising that multi-disciplinary opportunities are

not more widespread. Doubts remain about how far
such teams have been associated with changing
professional roles (Jefferys and Sachs, 1983). For
example, the majority of nurses attached to GPs are
district nurses and health visitors who are
employees of the local Health Authority. Although
working in part under the direction of the GPs,
there is no guarantee that these attachments promote
team care. Most surprisingly, practice nurses
constitute less than 10% of community nurses and the
potential for greatly increasing their numbers with
little, if any, cost to GPs has not been exploited
(Hart, 1985a; DHSS, 1986a). The possibility that
non-medical staff might also assume a wider range of
caring responsibilities in the PHC team has
sometimes materialised but most typically has not
(Dunnell and Dobbs, 1982; Bowling, 1985a).

While recognising some changes in the climate
of general medical services, an examination of the
experience of the health centre movement is
instructive of the difficult road to PHC in Britain.
One of the hopes expressed for the NHS in 1948 was
that their growth would be encouraged, yet by 1984
only about 25% of GPs were practising from them
(DHSS, 1984c). The supporters of the health centre
concept argued that it would generally improve the
quality of primary care, and more specifically would
enhance the growth of a team approach. The official
DHSS view was ambivalent, defining a health centre
as

> 'premises provided by an area health authority
> where primary health care services are provided
> for patients by general medical practitioners,
> health visitors and district nurses and
> possibly other professions' (HC[79]8).

The services offered would obviously vary, but it
was assumed that a basic range would include, in
addition to GPs, community nurses, ante-natal, pre-
school and school health, immunisation and
vaccination, and might extend further into dental,
hospital out-patient and various allied health
professional services.

The medical, and sometimes more general,
resistance to health centres has nowhere been more
evident than in the large conurbations. A recent
inquiry into the state of PHC in inner London
illustrated not merely the shortcomings of such
services as presently developed, but also the
growing pressure from financial problems confronting

the health services and the difficulties associated with unemployment and economic decline (LHPC, 1981, ch.1). London contains an especially high percentage of GPs working on their own and/or with a small list of patients. There is a marked lack of co-ordination between the hospital services and primary care, and a noticeable shortfall in resources for community, compared with hospital, services (chs.8-9). The LHPC report also expressed misgivings about the level of social and home support services (p.96). The general conclusion was of a frustrated, and at times beleaguered, PHC movement in the capital city.

Overall, the picture of PHC in the general medical services is of uneven and rather slow advances. Certainly there is evidence of progress, for example, with a more co-operative relationship among those involved with primary care. So too, more emphasis is being given to health prevention and promotion. But whatever the benefits for patients and GPs alike in such changes, they have not significantly modified the essential medical dominance of primary care (Noack, 1980).

Planning, Production and Management

How then has the health manpower process coped with the changing character of primary health care? As far as general medical practitioners are concerned the enhancement of primary care and of their role and status in the medical profession are very closely connected. In the early years of the NHS, there were grave doubts that GPs would survive the expansion and increased specialisation of hospital medicine. In the words of the then President of the Royal College of Physicians, GPs had 'fallen off the ladder' (Lord Moran, quoted in Watkin, 1978, p.44). Such dire prognoses proved unfounded, and the official embrace of primary care has given the general medical services a notable encouragement and enhanced standing.

Nevertheless manpower planning for GPs has remained a relatively under-developed art in comparison with hospital manpower. Imbalances in the supply of, and demand for, general practitioners have created far less political or professional comment - which appears paradoxical given that most illness is dealt with by the FPS rather than by hospitals. Consultants in tertiary care however have long enjoyed greater prestige and influence in health policy making. In increasingly cost conscious times planners' attention concentrates on the hospital services which consume the lion's share of NHS gross expenditure - 55.7% in 1951 rising to 62.0% in 1981, while the FPS proportion as a whole has fallen from 29.8% to 21.1% during the same period (Horder, 1985). Furthermore, the growing specialisation of hospital medicine has created particular problems for service planning, whereas general practice is much more amorphous in its skills and in the care expectations of patients.

Over the life of the NHS, GP numbers have increased in England and Wales from around 18,000 in 1949 to over 24,000 in 1980, with a further 3,000 in community and school health services. In comparison, doctors have almost trebled from 11,700 to over 31,000 whole time equivalents (BMA, 1983). This might be interpreted as a response to differential demand, but it is extremely difficult to draw easy conclusions about a shift between primary and secondary care on the basis of available health statistics. Horder (1985, p.55) examines selected aspects of the number of patients seen, or episodes of illness handled, as well as changes in the nature of the tasks undertaken across the two sectors and concludes that demand has moved unevenly, with trends favouring both general medical and hospital services.

Calculation of demand for GPs has therefore tended to stay 'safe' in doctor-to-population ratios, with an associated focus on the average list size. There has been a long term commitment both in the profession and the Health Departments to reduce the list size. In 1983 it stood at 2,081 in the UK, 2,116 in England, and 1,749 in Scotland (Dowson and Maynard, 1985). The objective of the BMA has been both to reduce the average list size to 1,700 and to impose some maximum figure. Table 8.1 shows the change in the size of GP practices in the UK during 1974 to 1983. A continued movement away from single handed practice is apparent (in 1952 43% of GPs worked in such a setting), and a tendency to work from a practice with four or more partners, 49% doing so in 1983. Such changes are partly a result of the official policy to reduce list size and partly of the encouragement to work within a health centre.

The maldistribution of GPs across the country has been an important factor justifying the increase in doctor numbers. There has been little attempt however to explore in detail whether maximum and minimum list sizes should be imposed, as indeed the

Table 8.1: Size of GP Practices in the UK, 1974-83*

Type of Practice**	1974 No	%	1983 No	%	% Change
Solo	4,505	18.0	3,508	12.3	- 5.7
2 Partners	5,359	21.5	4,792	16.7	- 4.8
3 Partners	6,333	25.3	6,399	22.3	- 3.0
4 Partners	4,484	17.9	5,671	19.8	+ 1.9
5 Or More Partners	4,319	17.3	8,271	28.9	+11.6
All GPs	25,000	100.0%	28,641	100.0%	+14.8

Source: Dowson & Maynard, 1985, Table 3

*   Figures for 1983 are estimates
**   Figures include some restricted principals in Northern
     Ireland and assistants in Scotland.

Table 8.2: Medical Practice Areas in England & Wales, 1974-81

Area	1974 % of GPs	av list size	1981 % of GPs	av list size
Restricted	13	1948	15	1889
Intermediate	39	2240	52	2101
Open	32	2478	32	2325
Designated	16	2722	1	2643
All	100	2355	100	2147

Source: Dowson & Maynard, 1985, Table 6

calculation of the demand for GPs has proven too complex in technical terms, and too enmeshed in strong professional interests. The Medical Practices Committees (MPCs) which must approve the appointment of GP principals in their Districts operate with classifications of areas as follows:

. restricted - an average list size of 1,700 or less;

. intermediate - 1,700 to 2,100;

. open - 2,100 to 2,500; and

. designated - 2,500 or more.

As can be seen from Table 8.2 such a policy would appear to have had some success, with the proportion of GPs working in 'designated' areas falling from 16% in 1974 to 1% in 1981. At the same time the proportion working in an 'open' area has remained constant. Given the overall aim of a list size of 1,700 there is still considerable room for change. As an estimation of demand average list size has limitations, not taking cognisance of a high proportion of the elderly or aspects of deprivation in the locality. Indeed, others, though not in a manpower context, have explored the issue of need for GP services, based on measures of workload (Jarman, 1983; Scott Samuel, 1984). Most importantly, the basic assumptions from which the MPCs operate, that GPs with low list sizes are looking for extra numbers, and that the whole population in an area is registered with a GP, do not hold in some places such as inner London (LHPC, 1981, ch.3).

The supply of GPs is usually linked with the same range of factors as outlined for their hospital counterparts (see Chapter 4). There is an important qualification however in that it is widely presumed that a medical student's career preference is to become a hospital consultant. Thus the rise and fall in supply of GPs is closely associated with the opportunities available in the hospital sector. The lower standing of general practice in the medical profession has been mentioned in this discussion, but there is some evidence of a changing perception. A mounting body of research (Parkhouse et al, 1983) indicates a gradual shift in career choice of medical students towards general practice. Horder (1985) reaches a similar conclusion: with 37% of

final year medical students reporting general
practice as their first choice in 1980 compared with
23% in 1966. The inference is that this trend
indicates a rising valuation and awareness of
primary care among medical students, as well as some
recognition of the diminished opportunities in
hospital medicine.

Aspiring GPs are not allowed simply to set
up practice as they wish. Where applications arise
from a vacancy in an existing practice, the MPC will
decide whether to authorise a replacement in
principle, and if so, will allow the remaining
partners to choose the successor. If the vacancy
occurs in a single-handed practice, the selection
process is the responsibility of the relevant FPC,
which makes a recommendation to the MPC, who
formally make the appointment. The MPC rejects
applications in 'restricted' areas and encourages
them in 'open' and 'designated' areas, as well as
offering special payments for practising in
'designated' areas. In 'intermediate' areas, each
application is considered on its merits (Dowson
and Maynard, 1985, pp.19-20).

Forecasting the demand for and supply of GPs
is therefore an extremely uncertain activity. Where
evident imbalances occur the formulation of plans
has relied on a mixture of positive incentives
rather than restrictive controls. This is
especially illustrated in the criteria for financing
general practice, and thereby affecting supply. It
extends well beyond support for setting up in under-
provided areas. Remuneration of general practice is
comprised of a range of allowances, reimbursements,
capitation and other items of service fees. These
fees are reviewed annually by the Doctors' and
Dentists' Remuneration Review Body (DDRB) which
makes recommendations to the Government.

> 'There has been some change in the relative
> career earnings of doctors in primary and
> secondary care in favour of the former, but not
> reaching parity' (Horder, 1985, p.66).

This may be a factor in increasing the supply of
GPs relative to hospital doctors, but most of the
evidence is anecdotal.

Remuneration for general practice has three
components:

　　1　Capitation Fees: an annual fee is paid for
　　　each registered patient depending on age;

in addition payment is made for out-of-hours services. These account for about 40% of a GP's income;

2   Allowances: a basic practice allowance is paid to each GP which can be supplemented: (a) if the practice is in a 'designated' area; (b) if it is a group practice; (c) to take account of the length of time a GP has practised; and (d) to allow for vocational training obtained and/or provided. On average, such allowances comprise 40% of a GP's income;

3   Item of Service Fees and Other Entitlements: a GP is entitled to a fee each time certain services are provided: for example, vaccinations and immunisations, cervical cytology, night visits, contraceptive services, and maternity medical services. Such fees account for about 18% of a GP's income (DHSS, 1986b, pp.56-7).

GPs are also reimbursed for practice expenses in terms of rent and rates, and as well as 70% of up to two ancillary staff salaries (p.58). Ancillary in this context includes receptionists, administrative and clerical staff, and practice nurses.

As with all of the health professionals surveyed, general medical practitioners have devoted a keen interest to problems of manpower production. At the undergraduate level there has been a growing input of primary care (Walton, 1985) but nothing comparable to the activity in improving postgraduate training for GPs. One sign of the progress made since the inception of the NHS is the elevation of the College of General Practitioners, which was founded in 1952 with the aim of improving the education and training of GPs, to the Royal College in 1969.

Prior to 1981 a physician who had completed the university medical degree and a pre-registration year in hospital(s), and became fully registered with the GMC, was entitled to enter general practice. A few general practices offered informal training schemes but the numbers involved were very small and it was widely seen as a means to gain prestige and lowly paid assistance for the senior partners. From the late 1960s onwards, rather more systematic, but still informal training was developed. The RCGP set out minimum standards for training and collaborated with Executive Councils (which pre-dated the FPCs) and Hospital Management Committees to design schemes which consisted of a prescribed combination of experience in appropriate hospital specialties and in general practice. The numbers going through such training before entering general practice increased sharply during the 1970s, and by 1981 covered some 70% of entrants.

In 1981 postgraduate training became legally compulsory for those setting up in general practice; for a transitional period one year's training was sufficient. The basis for certification is now three years' 'prescribed experience'. This includes one year as a trainee with a recognised GP trainer, and two years in an 'educationally approved' hospital or community medicine post, with 6 months each in two of the following specialties: General Practice, Geriatric Medicine, Paediatrics, Psychiatry, Accident and Emergency or General Surgery, Obstetrics and/or Gynaecology. To obtain certification, statements of satisfactory completion of the above posts have to be obtained and submitted to the Joint Committee on Postgraduate Training for General Practice (JCPTGP). The statutory regulations also provide for individual claims that experience outside the prescribed parameters is 'equivalent'. All NHS Regions offer formal GP vocational training schemes accredited by the JCPTGP, co-ordinated by Regional Advisors in General Practice, and by District GP course organisers.

The supply of trainees to such schemes is not calculated on any basis of required additions to the existing stock of GPs. There is some indirect regulation through controls over the number of recognised GP trainers. In addition, each trainer is allowed only one trainee at a time. However, GPs have a financial incentive to become trainers, with an allowance payable from FPC budgets. Certain standards have been set by the JCPTGP, and approval is initially for a probationary year in the first instance, and then at three yearly intervals. As it is not easy to withdraw the trainer status once granted, Regions have sought to deter unsuitable applicants. This concern with the approval of trainers and training practices has become a prominent aspect of recent campaigns and initiatives by the RCGP (1981; 1985) to enhance the quality of general practice (Schofield and Hasler, 1984).

The Royal Commission on the NHS Report (1979) identified three particular deficiencies in the training and management of GPs for their primary care activities: inadequate postgraduate training and performance review; the lack of national standards in the selection of principals in general practice; and problems of isolation and limited contact with professional colleagues (paras.7.29 - 31). The RCGP has identified similar problems:

'The opening up of general practice, the sharing of ideas and exposing different ways of practices, was something which touched only a small minority of doctors' (RCGP, 1985, p.1).

The RCGP has sought to improve the overall quality of GP vocational training and services with an emphasis on 'encouraging good practice' (DHSS, 1986b). The challenge is to the largely 'cherished individualism' which has virtually allowed practitioners to write their own job descriptions. Now the pressure is on GPs as a professional collectivity to put their own house in order before others do it for them.

Initiatives in health manpower management do not have to confront especially low job satisfaction, whereas there would appear to be scope for improvement of the 'level of competence and performance' (Fulop, 1980, pp.29-30). Balint's (1968) studies of general practitioners at work were a major stimulant to the RCGP sponsorship of inquiries on the subjects of what sort of doctor the profession was aiming for, and how GPs' performance might be assessed (RCGP, 1972; 1981). This appraisal has been paralleled in studies by the BMA through its General Medical Services Committee (GMSC). It has advanced six targets for improving general practice, which have direct implications for the delivery of primary health care (BMA, 1983).

The six targets are:

1 **personal care** - an acknowledgement that in many cases GPs do not devote sufficient time to patients. Although the GMSC does not indicate how this could be achieved, it is most likely to occur through a reduction in list size.

2 **the team** - this is regarded as a cornerstone of primary care and has the active encouragement of both the BMA and the Government. This is unlikely to reach desired levels given the present economic climate. With little resources

available on the DHA side for community health
services (the backbone of the team) it is
doubtful that many GPs would be willing to employ
their own resources as an alternative.

3 **service standards** - several factors are seen
as contributing to improvements in patient care
through recruitment, vocational training and
postgraduate training, along with a corresponding
reduction in patient list size from 2200 to 1700.

4 **balance of care** - an argument for a shift in
activities from the hospital sector to GPs, such
as minor surgery and paediatric surveillance.
There would have to be a concomitant transfer of
resources for this to become a reality, something
most DHAs are liable to resist given current
financial pressures.

5 **integration** - in the eyes of the GMSC the
independent nature of the GPs is an asset not a
liability to integration because it allows the GP
to take a broad perspective of patient needs.
This view is not without its critics who argue
that the very nature of GPs' independence is a
block on improving co-operation between the other
branches.

6 **accountability** - a recognition that GPs must
be held more accountable for the service they
provide, but not at the risk of jeopardising
their clinical role and responsibilities. It is
clear that interference in clinical matters will
not be tolerated yet to exclude this from any
accountability initiative inevitably weakens and
undermines the end result.

Few would dispute that these initiatives would
enhance and improve the quality of general practice
and benefit primary health care. The problem is
that for these proposals to become a reality would
require not only a transfer of resources from one
sector to another, but also a substantial increase
in the number of general practitioners.

The most recent discussion paper from the RCGP
(1985) indicates that some in its ranks are prepared
to adopt more explicit and stringent standards on
quality assurance. This elaborates four major
'areas of performance': clinical competence,
accessibility, ability to communicate, and
professional values. The objective is to establish

procedures for assessing experienced doctors under normal conditions which will stimulate improved quality of GP care. These proposals have attracted considerable criticism from within the profession (British Medical Journal, 5 October, 1985, pp.987-8; Campion, 1985) largely on the ground that remuneration should not be linked to quality of service and because of the general threat to the independence of individual doctors. Others pose a wider question: how far are GPs, for example, prepared to go in applying both stricter managerial criteria to their activities, as well as professional ones? For those concerned with the improved utilisation of the medical workforce, the focus on quality assurance is welcomed although doubts remain about the relevance of such an exercise to improving the efficiency and cost effectiveness of these medical services.

Fry (1983) offers a further perspective on reforming general practice, and with it primary health care. Improvements in clinical skills are emphasised along with ways of perceiving health and illness which are typically given prominence in treatises on PHC. More self-criticism among GPs is advocated and a greater readiness to engage in peer comparisons and practice reviews. He also advocates the promotion and development of the team approach to PHC, not just within the existing concept, but to experiment with and test out new roles and tasks. This could (and should) lead to a consideration of how many physicians, nurses, allied health professionals and other staff are really required. Finally, Fry extends this point into a criticism of national manpower policies, in particular suggesting that little has been done to discern 'how many general practitioners are really necessary' (p.79), while their numbers keep increasing year after year.

The concluding comments on the general medical services must then return to a now well-rehearsed argument that the organisational context in which health care is provided in Britain has inhibited service development outside the hospital sector. Furthermore, the planning, production and management of medical manpower has been a significant constraining factor. Progress has been slow and uneven in establishing medical manpower in the required numbers, and with the requisite skills and motivation. In addition, the financial resources made available to develop PHC are wholly inadequate (Green and Rathwell, 1985).

GENERAL DENTAL PRACTITIONERS

Since the establishment of the NHS, a majority of dental treatment has been provided by general dental practitioners (GDPs) who are administered by the family practitioner committees (FPCs) in England and Wales, but directly by Health Authorities in Scotland and Northern Ireland. There are in addition significant minorities on the Dental Register who are employed in: the community dental services (for pre- and school children, expectant mothers and those with a child under one year old, plus some handicapped adults); the hospital dental services; dentists employed by the armed forces; and those in private practice. Hospital and community dentists alone are employed by Health Authorities. Unlike the medical profession, this places the overwhelming proportion of dental officers in the category providing primary care (DHSS, 1983b).

When the NHS was first established, dentists' services were given free at the time of delivery, but charges were introduced in 1951 and have continued since then. The Dental Estimates Board (DEB) determines precise and maximum charges for the different courses of treatment, and dentists are then reimbursed on a fee-for-service basis by the DEB. The DEB monitors dentists' practices, and it can refuse payment on some more expensive courses of treatment where it deems the reasons unsatisfactory. Dental practitioners diverge even further from their medical counterparts in not operating with their own list of patients. Instead GDPs work on a 'course of treatment' basis to provide dental care, and after the service has been provided have no further formal connection with that individual, unless and until that person returns for a further course of treatment, when a new 'contract' is entered into.

Planning, Production and Management

Difficulties with the quite distinctive relationship between patient and dental practitioner have been widely voiced in recent decades (Royal Commission Report, 1979, ch.9). The fee-for-service method of payment, has hindered the meaningful promotion of dental health (Walker et al, 1965). The dental journals point to a number of major shortcomings as seen from their side. They claim that their remuneration is inadequate; that they are much constrained in their clinical freedom because of the restrictive application of the fee-for-service system; and that the dental profession has been forced into an unhappy compromise with demand for greater 'productivity' (ibid). According to the Royal Commission on the National Health Service Report,

'(g)iven the present level of disease and methods of practice, regular dental care can be given to considerably less than half the population. The fact that, in general, demand is much lower than need saves the service from breakdown' (para.9.14):

hence the regular complaints of a serious manpower shortage, and of the uneven distribution of practitioners across and within Health Authorities. In 1977, the number of persons per dentist ranged from 1 : 3,914 in England, to 1 : 4794 in Wales. This masked a considerable range: for example, from 1 : 2494 in the North West Thames RHA, to 1 : 5445 in the Northern RHA. Indeed, within the latter Region, there were further differences: with 1 : 3522 recorded in Newcastle and 1 : 7317 in nearby Sunderland (pp.106-7). The Royal Commission calculated that there would need to be a 60% increase in the number of dentists to bring the whole country up to the North West Thames figure.

Studies of dental manpower have appeared periodically over the last 40 years. A target figure of 20,000 active practitioners was recommended by the Teviot Committee in 1946 and this was reinforced by the McNair Report in 1956, although this set the 20,000 target for those on the Dental Register rather than the number in active practice. Recommendations were couched in terms of the poor dental health of the population and the unmet needs of those in the under-dentisted areas. The policy response favoured expansion of the dental school intake, and a figure of 954 per year was agreed in 1958, although not achieved until the mid-1970s. The target of 20,000 on the Dental Register was reached in 1978 (DHSS, 1983b). However, by this time the continued growth of the stock of dentists was increasingly being questioned - both within the profession and by government. A 10% cut in the intake of dental students in England and Wales was agreed for the mid-1980s, to bring recruitment to under 750 per year. As in medical manpower planning a general theme dominates the debates: what level of practitioners is compatible with attractive career prospects and rewards on the one hand, and reasonable dental fitness among the population on the other hand? If the immediate post-war years were pre-occupied with a perceived shortage of dentists, more recently fears are of a threatened over-production of staff in relation to effective demand and the financial constraints imposed on dental services.

This has created many difficulties and uncertainties for those attempting to forecast future requirements. Both the Royal Commission on the National Health Service, and the Nuffield Foundation Report on Dental Education (1980) felt uneasy about making firm policy recommendations. They cited the considerable problems in determining: the extent and treatment of dental disease; the productivity and work practices of GDPs; and the role of various assistants and auxiliaries. Nevertheless the forecasting nettle has been more firmly grasped in recent inquiries sponsored by the DHSS and the British Dental Association. In contrast to medical manpower, the Department and the profession both expressed optimism that manpower forecasting in dentistry offers greater prospects for success because '(d)ental needs are finite in a way that medical needs are not' (British Dental Journal, 1983, p.91; DHSS, 1983b, para. 1.7).

The current state of thinking on dental manpower is well illustrated in the report of the Dental Study Group on Dental Manpower (DHSS, 1983b), which includes the British Dental Association (BDA) report Dental Manpower Requirements to 2020 as an Appendix. There is a contrast in the methods employed for estimating demand and supply although both reports envisage a long term surplus of dentists. The BDA has taken the lead in measuring both the supply of, and demand for services in terms of 'courses of treatment'. It has broken with crude dentist-to-population norms as the basis for dental manpower planning, and instead focussed on the growth and distribution of the dentate and edentulous. This is supplemented by 'professional judgement' about dental care needs. In contrast the DHSS placed its main emphasis on estimating the size of the future dentate population and relating this to a demand for courses of treatment. It sought further evidence from regular surveys of dental health and people's inclination to seek dental care.

On the supply side, the central factors are listed as: treatment patterns (a presumed impact

172

from the fall in the incidence of caries in children); projections of the Dental Register (especially dental school output and the possible influence of migration); activity rates; dentists' productivity or treatment courses conducted; and the distribution of dental manpower (to under-provided areas) (p.120). Overall projections are rendered more problematic when estimates are formulated in terms of the main fields of practice in dentistry. For example, there is a specific issue over how much private practice is increasing among GDPs; and a further question mark is raised by the overlap in service between GDPs and the community service. The DHSS Study Group estimates a slight increase in the proportion in general practice over the period 1981 to 2020 from 78% to 81%, while those in secondary and supporting services will decline marginally (p.27). Even more difficulties surround forecasts about future treatment course content. While the dentate population is increasing, this adds to the number of teeth at 'risk' of treatment. More, but shorter, courses of treatment is the prediction.

It is on the basis of these main elements affecting the stock and flows of dentists that the 10% reduction in the undergraduate intake has been introduced, and with frank professional acceptance of the 'political' realities in dental manpower planning:

> '(t)here are dangers for the profession in overmanning, but patients suffer if there is undermanning. A fair balance has to be struck if a profession's overall political stance is to remain credible' (British Dental Journal, 1983, p.91).

Of equal moment is the professional relief that several areas of potential concern to dental practitioners have remained off the manpower agenda in these recent studies. Most notably, the DHSS Study Group felt able to assume that 'there will be no further delegation of major dental procedures to auxiliaries' (DHSS, 1983b, p.5). Issues of possible substitution were therefore completely shelved, but this replicated similarly dismissive comments in the Royal Commission Report (pp.114-5). At the same time the definition of need in projecting dental manpower requirements anticipates little divergence from current utilisation practices, while future supply is premised on existing productivity levels and little change in the organisation of services or the distribution of resources.

A major assumption underlying both the BDA and the DHSS approach to dental manpower is that the current imbalances in dental manpower and services will be corrected, although critics charge that this lacks a firm basis in detailed analysis (Birch and Maynard, 1985). Nevertheless it provides a rationale for the lack of service planning. Most significantly, and unlike GPs, dentists have been able to set up in practice without the approval of FPCs, and without vocational training and other (minimal) controls. Instead the major considerations are individual GDP preferences and market forces. Hence, for the vast majority of dental practitioners integration into wider NHS planning procedures seems even more in the distance than with their medical colleagues.

ADVANCING PRIMARY HEALTH CARE

However much primary health care in the NHS aspires to the ideals embodied in the WHO concept, in practice it is an often uneasy synthesis between those services provided by family practitioner committees - such as general medical and dental services - and the community health services of the DHA. For those in sympathy with the WHO assertion that 'health is a state of complete physical, mental and social well-being and not merely the absence of disease and infirmity' the aims and practices of the personnel and organisations in the non-hospital services seem limited if not misdirected. PHC in Britain has been following a narrow perspective and awaits the integration of community health services, family practitioner services, and other related non-NHS services.

Green and Rathwell (1985) postulate that in spite of known constraints a plausible and workable strategy for primary health care could be produced provided certain conditions are met. In order for the strategy to have any credibility FPCs and DHAs must co-ordinate their activities so as to:

. determine and agree, with the involvement of the community, specific health goals;
. create a climate for discussion by setting up mechanisms, either formal or informal, between providers, managers, and recipients of the services to debate policy initiatives;
. assess jointly the services currently available and discuss ways that such provisions could be

offered more effectively;
. recognise that in the short-term progress may only be possible through the DHA modifying or adapting its services in order to promote and foster closer links with those of the FPCs.

The link between performance and pay recommended in the recent RCGP (1985) consultation document has given the impression that even important medical opinion now acknowledges that established health practices may come under serious challenge. In an atmosphere which anticipates change (albeit 'reform or be reformed'), the terms of the PHC debate are being widened. For example, the local medical committee in Newcastle has produced a planning document which identifies five major problems in general practice -

'lack of direction, lack of accountability, poor measurement of outcome, inconsistency of service provision, and difficulty in reconciling the salaried community health service with an independent general practitioner grade' (Brown et al, 1986, p.371).

Their solution entailed making practices and not individual GPs responsible to the FPC for providing a guaranteed minimum of services in the acute, chronic and preventive fields. In the latter two areas, non-medical health professionals would play a much greater role than at present. Some staff currently attached to practices via DHAs might be contracted more directly in the general medical services (p.370-71). The Newcastle contribution is presented as one 'vision of the future' that stands besides the RCGP's quality initiative, and other schemes which 'range from the development of large group practices running a multiplicity of mini-clinics to use of nurse practitioners with general practitioners undertaking minor surgery' (p.371).
In contrast, the Government's Green (discussion) Paper Primary Health Care (DHSS, 1986b) indicates that those involved with policy formulation do not expect the present situation in the organisation and delivery of services to diverge greatly from what it is at present. In general terms, the health policy making agenda has been set by the central Health Departments' attempts to control NHS expenditure, and to focus attention on mechanisms to promote efficiency. Four themes were identified in the discussion paper:

'... to give patients the widest range of
choice in obtaining high quality primary health
care services;

to encourage the providers of services to aim
for the highest standards and to be responsive
to the needs of the public;

to provide the taxpayer with the best value for
money from NHS expenditure on the family
practitioner services;

to enable clearer priorities to be set for the
family practitioner services in relation to he
rest of the NHS' (pp.2-3).

Established service practices and manpower numbers
were not closely scrutinised, and utilisation
patterns and the skill mix of primary health care
workers remained unexplored. While the rhetoric of
the report mirrors the philosophy of HFA 2000, it is
short on detail and attention to issues of
implementation and evaluation. Established service
and manpower practices may thus be closely
scrutinised, and alternative modes explored. It is
against this context that Chapters 9 to 11 explore
three case studies of innovative manpower practices
in the primary health field.

Three general areas suggested themselves as
involving potential innovations on the manpower
front and with consequences for the development of
PHC. Firstly, following central Health Departments
priorities, the movement of hospital based services
into the community raises enormous planning and
implementation issues, including manpower aspects.
The area of mental handicap services was chosen as
the context of the first case study, in part because
of the intention to translate old manpower skills
into new and more appropriate ones for care in the
community. Focus lies on the approach adopted by
one Health Authority in South London.

A second area is that of the active pursuit of
PHC within the context of a purpose built health
centre. The contrast lies between a single handed GP
working only with, say, a receptionist and attached
community nurses, to a health centre, with a group
of GPs, receptionist, practice nurses, attached
community nurses, and other health related staff.
One health centre forms the basis of the second case
study. Interest lies in the manpower employed, the
general orientation to health care and their

patterns of teamwork.

The final choice lay with exploring emerging roles of staff working in the PHC context. Attention was drawn to the role of the nurse practitioner, working within an inner city general practice. Is this a new type of worker or an extension of the role of the nurse in general practice? It is the extended role of the nurse that forms the basis for the third case study.

Each of these case studies had within it the potential for a research project in its own right. Only a broad overview of the development, underlying philosophy central to the approach to provide primary health care, and the manpower dimensions were explored. Interviews were conducted with appropriate persons, as well as an attempt made to position the innovation, albeit briefly, within the context of relevant literature.

Chapter 9

FROM HOSPITAL TO COMMUNITY

The context for the first case study in relation to an 'innovative' manpower practice set out on lines consonant with HFA 2000 is the change in policy for the location of caring for mentally handicapped persons (Target 3, WHO, 1985b, pp.30-1). While the policy option is of considerable interest its manpower dimension is the focus of attention. The case study represents one District Health Authority's planning involvement in an aspect of primary health care and specifically the development of a community based, client centred mental handicap service. It demonstrates an attempt to plan and organise a service in which manpower is to be deployed according to the needs of the individual patients, and which by implication may challenge professional authority where this conflicts with patients' needs.

BACKGROUND TO THE POLICY OPTION

Services for the mentally handicapped in Britain have suffered from a legacy of Victorian attitudes and values. Care has been provided in early nineteenth century longstay hospitals often situated several miles from the nearest community. In effect, these acted as prisons, isolating, stigmatising and institutionalising their clients (Morris, 1969; Bayley, 1973; Mittler, 1979). Such a pattern of care also served to prevent the development or retention of skills which would enable them to live as 'normal' a life as possible in the community.

National policy for mentally handicapped persons is based on the principles outlined in the 1971 White Paper 'Better Services for the Mentally Handicapped' (DHSS, 1971). In particular, that document previsaged a major shift from institutional health service care for the mentally handicapped to a range of community care provided 'according to individual needs', and through the collaboration of local health and government authorities (especially social services). The Jay <u>Report</u> (1979) recommended a model of care where those mentally handicapped persons needing residential care away from home should receive it in small residential units, preferably in 'domestic housing' and sited in local communities. <u>Care in Action</u> (DHSS, 1981a) reiterated these principles, stressing the need for locally based services, planned jointly between local health and social services, with the close involvement of voluntary bodies and other agencies, such as education and training. The most recent statement of policy (DHSS, 1985b) reinforced this approach and responded to the critical review and evidence provided by the Social Services Committee of the House of Commons (1985b). Whilst such a policy applies across the United Kingdom, there are evident differences in emphases and implementation (Wistow, 1985).

Such a policy change of closing the large mental handicap hospitals and transferring care into the community, in locally based units or whatever, has enormous manpower implications in relation to the deployment of current staff, future recruitment, and basic and continuing education (Plank, 1982; Ferlie et al, 1984). Furthermore, the changes are '... dependent upon the provision of well planned services supported by multi-disciplinary teams consisting of practitioners of all disciplines involved with people who are mentally handicapped' (ENB, 1985b).

By far the largest group of NHS staff in direct contact with mentally handicapped persons is nurses. Such nurses are also specially qualified, having studied for a nursing qualification in mental handicap. The policy change thus has implications for the education and training of nurses. In 1982 a new syllabus for mental handicap training was proposed by the English National Board for Nursing, Midwifery and Health Visiting (ENB, 1982), a programme that is to be fully introduced in schools of nursing by 1987 (DHSS, 1985b). In addition, the ENB (1985b) has advocated updating the skills and knowledge of the 12,000 or so trained nurses, either state registered or state enrolled, caring for mentally handicapped persons.

The policy option of community care has not been without its critics. Three main questions have been raised. Firstly, the motivation of policy

179

makers and in particular the present Conservative
Government has been under suspicion. It has been
attacked for seeking to develop community care
solely from a belief that it provides a more
economic alternative to institutional care, while
also encouraging privatisation. In addition,
'community care' is seen as little more than an
ideological construct to reinforce the role of the
family, and specifically women, as the main carers
and units of support (Finch and Groves, 1980).
     Secondly, there is the issue of the resources
available for community care. Various interest
groups and critics have argued that in times of
financial cutbacks the pressure on both individual
carers and joint funding monies will lead to a
deterioration in support provided (Gladstone,
1982).

> 'You see, often parents see longstay
> institutions as wonderful because quite simply
> they have had such a raw deal from local
> authorities and the NHS, that is, no support
> basically. Convincing them that the services
> we will offer will be of value is particularly
> difficult'. *

     Thirdly, it is feared that either the community
will prove to be intolerant of mentally handicapped
people or mentally handicapped people themselves are
so severely handicapped that they cannot cope with
an independent life as they have been too
institutionalised to do so. A crucial issue is to
identify the needs of mentally handicapped people
and to relate these to an appropriate degree of
support, rather than economic considerations.

THE APPROACH ADOPTED

What then were the principles on which the DHA
developed a community based service, and how was the
closure of the District's longstay institution to
be managed? Within the District, prior to 1979,
services for mentally handicapped people were

---

* All quotations in this Chapter represent extracts
from interviews within the DHA unless otherwise
stated.

provided from an old Victorian longstay hospital.
It was in a serious state of delapidation to the
point where conditions were unacceptable both to
Government inspectors and to the local community
which was pressing for people not to be sent there.
The catalyst for generating action was a DHA
officer, who demonstrated a firm commitment to
develop mental handicap services. The problem
was defined initially by clarifying specific aims
and objectives for the clients. A report was
produced in 1981 for consultation within the Health
Authority, and formed the basis for the structure of
the service that was to be provided at a local
level.

The underlying philosophy of that report and
the proposed service, echoing the 1971 White Paper
and the Jay Report, was

'... based firmly on the belief and principle
that mentally handicapped people are equals in
their human value and rights with all other
citizens, and that mentally handicapped people
are developing human beings. Our fundamental
service principle is the principle of
normalisation'.

Thus the basic orientation was that every
handicapped person had a right to autonomy and
independence, and to a life within the community.
How then was this statements of rights translated
into service aims?

Three major avenues were pursued. Firstly, it
was argued that mentally handicapped people and
their families and friends must be involved in the
decision making processes 'from planning teams to
management committees and assessment boards', and
that, secondly, 'the most important needs of
mentally handicapped people are for other people not
buildings'. Thirdly, what became fundamental to the
service's development and form was the concept that

'when people have very special needs we should
look first at how we can bring extra resources
to them, rather than how we can bring them to
the services they need'.

The report commented that in the past clients had
suffered from fragmented and inadequately planned
services. There was a need for a long-term planning
approach and the adoption of an integrated model for
the development of services.

The structure of the new service involved the closure of the longstay institution and the movement of the patients into small houses which were either owned by local authorities, voluntary bodies, or mentally handicapped people themselves. The NHS would act as a transfer body. Support was to be provided on the USA model of 'care and cluster' houses. That is, there would be a care facility of a house, where a team of workers are based, who support a cluster of houses for clients. The social workers, psychologists, and so on would act as facilitators to normalise the mental handicapped person's environment. This approach aimed to de-institutionalise the patients; but it generated extensive debate about its feasibility for those who had been in an institution for anything from 10 to 30 years.

The closure of the longstay hospital began with an individual assessment of each client's abilities and needs. This assessment process involved a greater input than was originally thought necessary by officers as it took on average six months to a year to complete properly. It also became apparent that a shift away from the care and cluster model to a more individual approach was required. The service was set up by allocating people on a geographical basis. But,

'mentally handicapped people like everyone else don't make friends on a sector basis .... We had a very difficult time identifying, say, X authority people whose friends and relatives or people they are married to were not from another sector, and the NHS system is not flexible enough to take that on board'.

Inflexibilty over this issue originated from officers at both the DHA and at Regional levels, especially over funding: 'from the Treasurer's perspective the whole issue is system rather than people orientated'.

Another aspect with far reaching manpower implications was how the quality of service in the longstay hospital can be maintained as it is run down. The problem is one of coping in the interim while two forms of service, the old and the new, are in existence. These manpower implications were not addressed in 1981, but have since become a priority concern:

'at the moment we have a clear division of

ideology and practices between the new community and residual hospital services, with a great deal of antipathy between those two groups'.

Morale among staff in the longstay hospital is very low and a 'brain drain' has occurred whereby good staff and management have transferred out of the service because they see no future for their careers.

Moreover, finding a means of defining the exact skills that will be required for the new service has proved difficult. The officers involved have attempted to evaluate the skills which can be carried over. This has been particularly contentious as the fundamental aim of the new service is to de-professionalise care as far as possible. It is the DHA's belief that

'any professional and systematic service input into mentally handicapped services is stigmatising and is a non-normal environment .... The basic philosophy is that a mentally handicapped person is no different from the rest of us, and if they need specialist skills then they need specialist skills, but not first because they are mentally handicapped'.

The community based manpower requirements will make most medical staff for the mentally handicapped obsolete as well as extensive numbers of psychologists and nurses whose skills are deemed inappropriate for community based care. Certainly the Authority recognises that some mentally handicapped people will require psychological and psychiatric care, but they reject the idea that is put forward by the professions that all clients need regular assessment. Not surprisingly, workers and professionals in mentally handicapped services saw the changes as an attack on professional control and authority.

At one level, health care practitioners have reacted to fears about job security, an issue which has only slowly been recognised as a valid concern by management. In the early stages of the service development, the manpower implications did not figure prominently. However, the Authority has lately identified the need to set aside 1-2% of the revenue budget for training and retraining of manpower. It also plans to reduce significantly its allocation to the acute sector over the next 10 years and expand community care services accordingly. Thus,

> 'the unions are legitimately going to argue, well you can't make our members redundant and then appoint other people. What prospect is there for transfer and retraining? As yet our Authority hasn't got an answer for that, and I don't think anywhere has as yet in the Health Service'.

The Authority has still to identify the manpower skills which will be needed to support an autonomous and independent existence by mentally handicapped people. Professionals claim a degree of occupational autonomy in order to sustain their status and authority; management has found this directly conflicts with their perception of the needs and requirements of the client.

> 'The professions themselves are the biggest hurdle you have to overcome. It doesn't matter what standards or objectives and philosophy you adopt, they all become moulded by the professions to fit their own ends'.

The input of such professionals was however needed by those who had been resident for a lengthy period in the longstay institution because of the extensive erosion of the clients' social skills; but now it is deemed essential to develop a less professionally structured environment.

Who then will be these new community based workers and what expertise will they need? The aim of the Authority is for the service to be predominantly run by a very few managers and 'non-professional' staff, with some more specialised staff to undertake skills training of the mentally handicapped. An attempt is being made with local authorities and voluntary organisations to establish orientations towards caring which do not depend on existing professional roles.

> 'The workers will be a paid carer who will make sure that skills which have been learnt were being retained (for example, that people got up, made their breakfast, etc), that the basic level of care is being maintained and then they act as a danger light who can identify when problems occur and then at the second level bring in more specialised care'.

But their job is also one of eliminating the need for regular psychiatric and psychological care, which is perceived as being not only unnecessary, but also stigmatising and a means of preventing the mentally handicapped from developing a 'normal' life.

'In the field of community handicapped services these workers see their role as providing the young and adolescent handicapped with an umbrella which keeps the NHS and local authorities off the mentally handicapped person's back, and which allows them to develop in as free an environment as possible'.

The position of the nursing workforce is at yet unclear. Some of the newcomers will be nurses who have embraced an interdisciplinary role.

'The nurses will either de-professionalise themselves and become new mental handicap workers in the community, or they will slide backwards into type and fight to keep the long-stay institutions open. It is unclear which way that is going to go'.

However, in the main the role of the new worker is envisaged as reducing the mystique surrounding the professional care of the mentally handicapped. Management has also had to develop new skills and abilities. It has had to develop means of smoothing the transfer of the mentally handicapped back into the community and overcome community antagonism to such a move, a hostility which the Authority did not anticipate. However, groundwork by both the Authority officers and the Community Health Council managed to sway local public opinion in favour of the plans for the new community based service. The pressure from individual Authority members was to a large extent responsible for generating both the initial impetus for the project, as well as seeing it through to the formulation of official policy.

CONCLUSION

Key individuals within an organisation such as the NHS can often act as pivotal or focal points for developing or blocking changes to service provision. The example of this Health Authority provides a further illustration:

> 'The lesson is very much that it doesn't matter
> what system you adopt, if you don't have the
> right people in the right place you won't get
> anywhere. We (in Britain) have been talking
> for 20-30 years about closing longstay
> institutions and it was never going to happen
> ... Since X ... and Y ... came here we (the
> DHA) are two years away from that'.

While the services for the mentally handicapped had
to be replanned on the lines of Government
priorities, the exact form, timing and enthusiasm
were thus significantly affected by a committed
individual(s). Joint funding acted as an additional
stimulus.

In terms of the manpower implications of the
policy, the management dimension is clearly to the
fore - namely, how to provide jobs for the current
workforce, and how to provide appropriate personnel
for the caring role in the community - whilst the
planning and production aspects are close behind -
where to recruit the appropriate persons for the new
hostel-like facilities, and future training and
continuing education. It is a moot point as to
whether those employees who are used to working in a
longstay institutional environment possess the
necessary skills or commitment for a community role.
It is also problematic as to whether current staff
can be retrained, or whether a 'new' type of worker
has to be produced. If the latter option is pursued
the present workforce will have to be redeployed,
with implications for training and teamwork.

This case study presents the approach pursued
by one Health Authority. As the DHSS (1985b) have
pointed out, there are

> '... still nearly 70 mental handicap hospitals
> in England with over 200 beds, and nearly 50
> with between 100 and 200. An estimated minimum
> of 9,000 hospital residents could live outside
> hospital immediately if alternative
> accommodation was available' (p.49).

Many other DHAs are thus having to face a similar
problem. In each, the needs of the client group
(whose requirement in general is for social not
medical care), of the current workforce (a range of
professionals anxious over their own jobs, and over
their professional status and authority), and of the
future workforce (a more caring role) are the
primary challenges to be addressed.

As to the success of the policy option, it has established the philosophy that mentally handicapped persons should be allowed and have a right to live as normally as possible. However, it requires the injection of sufficient financial and personnel resources, which is problematic. More broadly, success has to be judged in terms of an improvement in the quality of the service and the quality of life of the clients. The Authority is seeking to develop a means of measuring quality and in particular, of eliciting the views of the mentally handicapped people themselves, but its exact form remains to be clarified.

'It worries me. How do we go about monitoring quality in the community? .... We don't yet know for sure that having someone in a DHSS house with community care is better'.

Chapter 10

PRIMARY HEALTH CARE IN ACTION

The growth of health centres in Britain has only
assumed any real significance since the 1960s,
although the health centre ideal has a long if
checkered history. It has been variously
interpreted and championed. In recent years it has
been increasingly advocated as an essential
component of primary health care. But a question
mark remains about the extent to which the majority
of health centres existing within the NHS were
established with a wide-ranging PHC role in mind.
The discussion in this Chapter begins with a brief
overview of the context in which health centres have
developed in Britain, and then focusses on one
attempt to put the theory of PHC into practice.

Health centres first achieved official
recognition in the Dawson Report of 1920. This had
been set up to advise the Minister of Health on 'the
ideal system of medical and allied services' (quoted
in Honigsbaum, 1979, p.64). Dawson himself
initially conceived of health centres as collective
surgeries, but he subsequently argued for a more
extended notion where general practitioner (GP),
hospital and local authority services were housed
under the same roof. The proposal was not a
straightforward initiative to improve health care,
but was also stimulated by a desire to give greater
unity to the medical profession (p.106). Other
medical reformers, such as the State Medical Service
Association, advanced variations on this model. The
support generated for health centres could not
however overcome the suspicion in government
circles, and the marked hostility from important
sections of the medical profession. There were
particular qualms that the introduction of health
centres would heighten conflicts between GPs and
consultants. More generally, there was a
suspicion that the health centre was the thin end of

the wedge of state medicine and a salaried medical
service. The only serious attempt to implement such
a scheme was undertaken at the Pioneer Health Centre
in Peckham - first between 1925 and 1930, and then
more ambitiously from 1935 (Pearse and Crocker,
1943). The Peckham experiment highlighted health
rather than illness services. It emphasised an
active rather than a passive involvement in healthy
living, and put the family and environmental issues
to the fore. It also presumed a more significant
role for the general practitioner. However, it
failed to inspire a wider movement within the
medical profession, and even among the general
public there was little obvious appreciation for
this initiative (Lewis and Brookes, 1983).

Evidence that the health centre ideal had not
been lost was signalled in the National Health
Service Act (1946) which contained a provision for
its development on a nationwide basis. Little
immediate progress followed the inception of the
NHS, although by the mid-1960s the Ministry of
Health reported that the long term plans of local
Health Authorities revealed an upsurge in interest.
In March 1965, 36 centres were identified, and this
was expected to grow to 284 by March 1976, with one
quarter planned for the London area (Ministry of
Health, 1966, p.6). The Royal Commission on the NHS
Report (1979) suggested that the expansion had taken
place - with 212 in 1972 and a projection of 731 for
1977 in England and Wales. Scotland and Northern
Ireland seemed even better provided, although there
were complaints that the growth in urban areas, and
especially London, had not been achieved (paras.
7.48-49).

These figures suggest a marked departure from
the traditional pattern of general practice,
although the term health centre has not been
consistently defined by the central Health
Departments. In Kohn's (1983) comprehensive review,
it can be understood:

> 'first as a physical facility accommodating
> the health team and its equipment, and second
> as an administrative concept encompassing any
> arrangement whereby a variety of services are
> integrated to provide comprehensive primary
> care'(p.22).

The Ministry of Health had sponsored health centres
as a means of encouraging GPs to set up practice in

'under-doctored' areas, especially where the cost or suitable location of premises would create difficulties, as in inner London. An important attraction for GPs to set up in health centres has been the financial inducement since the capital investment is already provided, as are rental charges, although the GP must bear the running costs. The stimulus to extend and enhance the services to patients has been less obvious.

This official viewpoint is further reinforced in the restricted definitions of health centres offered. The Ministry of Health (1966) referred to:

'premises which combine facilities for general practitioner and for local authority services, and sometimes include consultant out-patient facilities'.

A decade later, the DHSS (HC(77)8) view had not expanded significantly:

'premises provided by an Area Health Authority where primary health care services are provided for patients by general medical practitioners, health visitors and district nurses and possibly other professions'.

Later in the same document, however, it is recognised that a health centre may incorporate a much wider range of family practitioner services, allied health professionals and health related services.

The Royal Commission on the NHS Report (1979) regarded this breadth of interpretation of the health centre concept as a virtue, and argued against forcing general practice 'into one particular mould' (para. 7.51), even if this fosters examples which do not correspond closely to currently favoured designs for PHC. In consequence the British experience of health centres spans a continuum from minimal GP and attached nursing services, to a broad based primary health care team, with innovative ideas in terms of practitioners' roles, patient involvement and general approach to health care. In the case study which follows, the clear possibilities for exploring PHC in a health centre environment are illustrated.

A HEALTH CENTRE: POTENTIAL AND PRACTICE

The health centre is situated on the outskirts of a
northern industrial city, in a predominantly working
class catchment population of 10,000 which like the
city as a whole has a high level of unemployment. It
is a purpose-built facility provided and maintained
by the DHA. At the time of interview there were
about 40 paid workers including administrative and
clerical staff (Table 10.1). In addition, there
are a number of voluntary workers who run the
patients' library and the Citizens Advice Bureau.
The majority of employees are employed by the GPs
via the FPC remuneration scheme, with the DHA
employing the attached health visitors and district
nurses. The social worker is attached to the health
centre which is a cause of some misgivings:

> 'we have I think really lost out there as we
> really don't get any feedback' (Occupational
> Health Worker).

A counsellor's post also exists but was vacant.
The centre has initiated two notable
developments aimed directly at generating greater
accountability to patients and other health workers.
These are the management committee and the patient
participation group. The management committee was
set up with the intention that it would make all the
policy decisions concerning health care. All
workers are represented on it, including domestic
and clerical staff. It consists of one member from
each of the different occupational groups, as it was
felt essential that no interest group was over-
represented, and that all workers had equal decision
making power. The majority of staff indicated that
decisions regarding the policies of the centre were
negotiated, although some problematic areas were
identified. For example, the nurses were employees
of the GPs and so complete equality in decision
making was inhibited at times. Notwithstanding, a
more participatory process was evolving.

> 'Yes, but often reservations towards new ideas
> do come through on the basis of old hierarchies
> but it is really changing with the setting up
> of the health food shop, our newest venture.
> It was the most broad based initiative we have
> made here ... and, the most widely supported
> and agreed upon one' (Occupational Health
> Worker).

191

Table 10.1:   The Health Centre's Staff

8 receptionists and clerical staff
7 doctors (3 female)
5 community psychiatric nurses
3 community nurses - health visitors and district
  nurses
2 health visitors
2 nurse practitioners (geriatric and preventive
  care)
2 occupational health workers
2 unemployment and health workers
2 workers for the mentally infirm
1 chiropodist
1 community midwife
1 counsellor (vacant)
1 foot care assistant
1 dietary nursing assistant - running the
  wholefood shop
1 health visitor for geriatric patients
1 patient liaison officer
1 social worker

Note: The job titles are as designated within the
Health Centre.

The patient liaison officer is a member of
the management committee, as well as being the
chairperson of the patients' participation group.
The specific role of this officer is to act for the
patients and to bring forward and act upon their
problems or criticisms. The aims and areas of
involvement of the patients' participation group are
more ambitious:

> '(to) encourage patients to take on active
> roles in determining what health care is
> offered rather than the normal state of affairs
> where the "patient" passively accepts whatever
> the doctor doles out'.

Patient participation groups are a new development
to family practitioner services, and have only
existed since 1972, with the National Association
for Patient Participation in General Practice being
set up in 1978. The number of such groups still

remains small (70 in total) with the vast majority
of those in existence having been set up by the GPs
rather than the patients. The philosophy behind
such groups is that doctors and patients work
equally together to improve services and to
stimulate greater awareness of patients needs and
reactions, while encouraging patients to greater
self-understanding about their own health and
organisation of care.

The health centre's group was set up in 1976
with the initial stimulus coming from one of the
GPs. The group's membership is automatic for
everyone registered as a patient at the centre.
The broad aims of the group are as follows:

'to give patients a say in running
the health centre; to improve communication
between doctors, health workers and
patients, and to provide feedback from
patients to all the health workers at the
centre; to provide a way of dealing with
suggestions and complaints; to promote health
education; to support ways of increasing
the active participation of patients in the
management of their own illnesses; to
provide a base for voluntary community care;
and to campaign for better provisions of health
services and improvements in the level of
care available'.

It has been recognised that in order to fully
develop a community based service which 'responds
to the expressed health needs of the community'
(WHO, 1978), it is essential to formalise its
particiption.

'If you are going to keep a health centre to
advantage patients, then they have got to
be brought into the formal structures in a
formal way, to get other health workers to see
that they are an essential part' (GP).

This policy has been actively supported in the
centre.

'The Patients' Association is a great advantage
to us, because it allows us to see how we are
doing and the mismatch between how we think
we are doing and how well we are in fact
doing' (Occupational Health Worker).

However, the staff acknowledged that conflicts have arisen. One example which had to be resolved was the demand for the patient liaison officer to be on the management committee. This was eventually agreed.

What then has the Patients' Association achieved? It has been taken into the formal decision making process of the centre, and its suggestions tended to be acted upon. The group championed the appointment of three women GPs, so that women patients had a choice over which doctor they consulted. Also the Patients' Association has become involved in numerous projects, and has provided a range of new services and facilities. Its members run health education lectures, keep fit classes, and purchase equipment such as home blood sugar and pressure meters. The group has also set up or provided the initial stimulus for three projects which are important for the development of an educative and holistic approach to health care. These are the setting up of a Citizens Advice Bureau (CAB), a patient's library and a health food shop at the centre. The CAB is staffed by trained volunteers from the advice organisation, and provides a confidential social advice service one evening a week, dealing primarily with social welfare and personal problems. The patient's library operates from the waiting room and has 200 books available for loan on various aspects of health care. The library is staffed by volunteer members of the Patients' Association. The waiting room itself is also organised by the Patients' Association and is strikingly different from most GPs' surgeries, with its comfortable chairs, coffee, the showing of health videos, and a children's play area.

A health food shop has been recently set up on the premises which provides the local community with easy access to health foods. The shop is staffed by a dietary nursing assistant who provides patients with advice on nutrition and diet.

'On the food front we as health workers were acutely aware of a lack of any real input into diet and felt it was useless telling people to change their diet without providing any real support for that' (GP).

The fundamental aim of the centre has been to

'integrate population based preventive care
with curative care, taking as your base point
the whole individual' (GP).

The underlying philosophy is one in which the
individual seeking health care is not perceived as a
passive patient, but a participant working with the
professionals towards promoting health. In order to
establish such an approach and integrate preventive
and curative work, the health centre established
priorities for change. One of the first areas they
identified was the need to reduce patient-doctor
ratios as it was felt that the time allowed for
consultations was crucial to improving doctor-
patient relationships, and to providing any form of
educative or preventive care service.

'It is no good having all these innovations and
ideas if you're still working on the old
calling shop mentality' (GP).

It was argued that a patient should have at least
a ten minute consultation and the doctor a patient
list of not more than a thousand. As a way of
achieving this the number of GPs at the centre was
raised from four in 1977 to seven by 1985. However,
such an expansion created its own difficulties.

'The problem is in the present system because
maximum remuneration is given to those who
spend the least on additional resources and who
have the highest patient list, so (there is) a
disincentive to improve care. To get ours to
seven (GPs) has been a major fight. As soon as
it affects income ideas go out of the window'
(GP).

In order to integrate preventive and curative
care it was felt necessary to reject traditional
roles and responsibilities for health workers, and
to adopt a team based approach. There were, at the
time of the interview, five nurses based at the
health centre, three of whom were community nurses
employed by the Health Authority and accountable
to the Director of Nursing Services for the
Community. This situation was perceived to be
unsatisfactory as the health centre had no
involvement in deciding how many community nurses
worked from it, or even over who they were. On one
occasion these nurses had been changed on what
appeared to the centre to be an arbitary basis,

with only 24 hours notice.

The other two nurses are employed by the GPs. These nurses describe themselves as nurse practitioners (NPs). Neither wears a uniform, and patients can self refer to them as well as be referred by the GPs. They argue that the nursing input they provide is fundamentally important within general practice: delivering a service on a nursing, rather than a medical model, where preventive and educative community based work can easily be rooted. In addition, in terms of their clinical practice, both NPs are described as 'autonomous practitioners', in that they are responsible for consolidating and developing a role, which rests on identifying and responding to a patient's needs without necessarily prior consultation with a GP.

Each nurse practitioner works with specific groups of patients. One is a preventive care nurse with responsibilities for initiating and running a well-woman clinic, which includes a cervical and a cardiovascular screening clinic. Her aim is to increase people's knowledge of and control over their own health status.

> 'Patients who visit this nurse are educated and advised about how best to change their lifestyle to improve their blood pressure. The choice is then theirs. If such advice is taken but fails to reduce the person's blood pressure, then drug therapy is maybe used as a last resort'.

The second nurse practitioner works with the elderly in the community as well as in the surgery, providing a first point of contact for those who have simple health problems or whose needs require support and counselling rather than medical input. Her work is again educative and preventive. Due to the high proportion of home visits that she makes she is well placed to identify potential health problems before they become critical and refer the patient on to the GP.

The centre has developed two other initiatives for elderly people in the area, which complement the work done by the NP. The first of these is the Elderly Mentally Infirm project, initially funded by MIND. The project employs two workers who describe themselves as 'non-professionals', as well as several volunteers. They utilise their extensive local knowledge and in a largely supportive role visit the elderly confused regularly in their own

homes, providing practical help to their carers.
This often takes the form of simply listening and
talking to the old person, or providing an
opportunity for the carers to go out. Thus these
workers try to sustain the informal family care
system and to prevent the health, both physical and
psychological, of the carers from deteriorating. A
further aim is to refer the elderly to non-medical
staff such as the NP, or the social worker. The
second initiative is that of a specialist health
visitor for the elderly who was funded initially
as a one year pilot scheme. The main involvement of
this health visitor is the running of a weekly
Retirement Clinic. Its aim is to provide support in
encouraging elderly people to pursue and maintain
their social activities before retirement causes
isolation and loss of self-esteem. Thus the health
visitor sees her most important role as enabling
elderly people to identify their own needs and
requirements and not to simply accept other people's
definitions.

Without further research and analysis it is
difficult to determine the success of these service
initiatives, or to what extent the nurses are
autonomous practitioners. But the centre has made
positive attempts to develop the role of the
nurses, to make better use of their skills and
approach to care. One move in support of their
autonomy has been for the management committee,
rather than the GPs, to control the nurses. Thus
although the nurses' posts are funded on the FPC
reimbursement scheme, their channel of
accountability is through the management committee.

'The nurses have got a defence structure ...
and aren't under the thumb of the doctor. If
the doctors perceive the role of the nurse as
syringing ears, they have to negotiate that
through all the committees here' (GP).

However, problems have been identified in this
process of change. The nurses found that self
referral by patients was very low initially; the
preventive care nurse found that it was only after a
period of six months that her clinics really began
to establish themselves with patients. Existing
working practices and hierarchies proved resistant
to change.

'Traditional values die hard and if people are
insecure about these new open structures, which

197

they are, then they will be bypassed and old hierarchies will re-emerge' (GP).

A further important project to be initiated at the health centre was one relating to occupational health. Estimates of industrial disease and occupationally caused ill health are a matter of dispute (Doyal and Epstein, 1983). The NHS has failed to respond to this problem area. A pilot study was set up over three years ago with another GP practice in the city. Its aim was to provide a means for general practice (and PHC) to respond to occupationally generated ill health, and to incorporate a means of preventing work-related illness. Four workers are employed. The project staff operate at two levels. Firstly, they interview patients at the health centre about their work history in order to correlate symptoms with known work hazards and inform both patient and GP. Secondly, the project has aimed to address the causes of industrial disease. This is approached from a community health position rather than individual cases. The project's employees therefore conduct meetings to educate workers and trade unions about health threats, and leaflet the local community. Thirdly, they campaign for known hazards to be removed from local workplaces, through changes in production processes or through greater workers' self-protection. For example, a successful campaign has been waged for a local firm to cease using products which had been causing dermatitis among the centre's patients. Linked to this project, the centre is setting up an 'unemployment and health project' to strengthen and develop awareness about links between unemployment and ill health. The unemployed in the area were felt to be particularly isolated, given the location of the practice population which is some distance from the city centre. Both projects also act as referral points passing people on to other more appropriate health workers or voluntary agencies such as the Citizens Advice Bureau or community psychiatric nurses.

CONCLUSION

The potential that health centres offer for providing an environment in which primary health care consonant with the aims espoused in HFA 2000 may flourish has been widely noted. The Royal Commission on the National Health Service Report (1979), and the Harding Report (1981) both reflect the mounting support for teamwork in primary care. Not only is the health centre a catalyst to a changing division of labour in health care, but a stimulant to greater emphasis on health prevention and promotion services. The experience to date has been mixed. The organisation and delivery of services from health centres varies considerably, and doubts linger whether more than a minority have lived up to the high expectations of their advocates (Cartwright and Anderson, 1981; Jefferys and Sachs, 1983; Ruston, 1985).

The evaluation of health centres is far from straightforward in large part because there is a wide interpretation of their key elements. Nowadays 'teamwork' has become 'the talisman of experiment and progress in the organisation of health services' (Reedy, 1980, p.108). The predominant view in official reports has been that the character of teamwork generated in the hospital and primary care settings is quite different. In the former, the emphasis is on medical rather than health care, with professional roles more clearly defined and hierarchical. In contrast, PHC objectives are both more comprehensive and less focussed, and medical dominance of other practitioners less certain (Hicks, 1976; Reedy, 1980). The PHC team has more scope for flexibility in its service roles and health objectives. In Reedy's (1980) terminology it has both 'centripetal' and 'centrifugal' functions; it acts both as a gatekeeper as well as a 'case finder' and facilitator of an improved awareness of health. Notwithstanding, so much discussion is premised on a minimal link between health care professionals as being sufficient to constitute teamwork: for example, those schemes which attach nurses to GPs.

The growth of genuine multi-disciplinary teams has therefore depended less on Health Authorities than on the understanding and enthusiasm of the professionals themselves. A study of a group practice in Cleveland concluded that where professional sympathy and involvement existed there were grounds for optimism (Marsh and Kaim-Caudle, 1976). GPs, nurses and patients alike all expressed general satisfaction with the way in which the nurse contribution to care had been enhanced. Gilmore et al's (1974) investigation of nurse attachment schemes illustrated how widely practice varied in the implementation of teamcare beyond basic contact in their working from the same base. Bond et al (1985) concluded in a similar fashion that the concept of 'teamwork' is best replaced by 'interprofessional collaboration'.

Interprofessional collaboration entails a broader perspective of joint working. It builds on a taxonomy suggested by Armitage (1983):

1 Isolation - members who never meet, talk or write to one another;

2 Encounter – members who encounter or correspond with one other but do not interact meaningfully;

3 Communication - members whose encounters or correspondence include the transference of information;

4 Collaboration between two agents - members who act on that information sympathetic- ally; participate in patterns of joint working; subscribe to the same general objectives as others on a one to one basis in the same organisation;

5 Collaboration throughout an organisation - organisations in which the work of all members is fully integrated.

(Bond et al, 1985, Table 1.4 - based on Armitage, 1983)

In their own research based on this schema, Bond et al (1985, ch. 12) report that the majority of their nurse respondents could be placed in the 'isolation', 'encounter' and 'communication' categories. The minority fitted the 'collaboration' stages; they were more noticeable among district nurses (about 25%) than among health visitors (around 10%), although less than 5% in both cases reported 'full collaboration'.

The health centre examined in this case study appears to be operating along the lines of 'full collaboration' as described by Armitage (1983). Although in the research project a quantitative record of working practices was not attempted those interviewed expressed general agreement that the centre had made important strides towards inter- professional collaboration. Most of the staff were fully aware of the aims underlying joint working and were committed to their enhancement. A range of informal and formal structures facilitated close

working relations between staff, as well as with
patients. This health centre sought an especially
ambitious professional collaboration which extended
beyond innovation in manpower utilisation to
encompass supportive practices in community health
promotion and prevention. The revamping of
professional roles was directed to mounting a
challenge to the sexual division of labour in health
care and the downgrading of women's health issues
and interests. These developments were viewed as
part of a wider endeavour to address economic,
social and occupational factors in ill-health while
also responding to the individual client's health
needs.

Nevertheless points of tension and conflict
still emerge. Not all staff shared the same
enthusiasm for full joint working, or a move towards
the notion of 'equal partners'. The attachment of
nurses was a special area of concern since the
health centre had no control over which staff
worked from their premises. This example of a
health centre highlights the ways in which the
'established' organisation of health manpower
planning, production and management may disadvantage
innovatory practices. In particular, there are few
incentives which encourage full inter-professional
collaboration. The extension of professional
enthusiasm for such schemes is therefore most
problematic. The health centre occupies an uneasy
position between the Health Authority and the FPC.
Without the unambiguous backing of health planners
even the most innovative primary health care team
will find itself frustrated. It is a sad commentary
on the NHS that a health centre which provides
health care along lines supportive of HFA 2000 is so
atypical.

Chapter 11

EXPANDED ROLE FOR THE NURSE OR NEW WORKER?

INTRODUCTION

In the 1960s a new primary health care role was
evolving in North America, namely that of a 'nurse
practitioner'. The nurse once given suitable extra
training in the areas of physical assessment,
diagnosis and treatment would act as a 'physician
extender' (Stilwell, 1982b), and fill a gap in
health care provision in so called 'under-doctored'
areas, in outlying rural districts and inner city
zones. Since that time, the nurse practitioner role
has undergone codification, many variations in
working relationships with primary physicians have
been established, and numbers increased, 15,000 or
so now practising (Draper, 1981). Some nurse
practitioners work in 'autonomous' practice outside
the direct supervision of a physician; others in
'semi-autonomous' practice, where there is easy
access to physician opinion but the nurse does not
work as a team with the physician; yet others in
'collaborative' practice where the nurse
practitioner and physician work as a partnership,
referral between the two being easy and usual
(Stilwell, 1982c, p.1909).
    The scope of practice of the nurse practitioner
in the USA has been summarised as follows (Stilwell,
1982a, p.1800):

.   to assess the physical and psychosocial health
    status of patients;
.   to discriminate between normal and abnormal
    findings from screening;
.   to evaluate diagnostic data collected and decide
    on treatment either independently or with a
    physician;
.   to manage patient care within protocols mutually

> agreed by medical and nursing personnel, including prescribing and adjusting medication;
- and, to lay emphasis within each patient consultation on developing a relationship which is conducive to health promotion.

It can thus be seen that a new type of worker in primary health care as an aide or assistant to the primary physician has developed, but built upon elements within the nursing process, particularly the concern with the physical, mental and social status of patients and a counselling and guidance role.

It was against this background that a scheme was developed in a Birmingham inner city practice to establish and evaluate the contribution of a 'nurse practitioner' role to primary health care. After a period of further training, acquired through apprenticeship to a general practitioner (GP), full-time nurse practitioner services were offered to patients in January 1981 (Stilwell, 1982a). It is this innovative manpower practice that forms the focus of the third case study. After exploring aspects of its workings the innovation is set in a wider context of the role of nurses in general practice.

THE BIRMINGHAM PROJECT

Stilwell (1982a) outlines the aims of the nurse practitioner (NP) project (1981-85) as follows:

- to extend the services already available in the practice by providing more consultation time for patients, as well as offering health maintenance, and the educative facilities of the NP's consultations;
- to teach the patient to take more responsibility for his/her health;
- to offer a less formal style of consultation which might encourage the patient to share problems or anxieties which may, directly or indirectly, affect health (p.1801).

The General Practice Teaching and Research Unit of the University of Birmingham was responsible for the evaluation of the project. Four aspects were examined:

- the acceptability of the extended role of the nurse in a general practice setting, to patients and to other health practitioners;
- the motives and expectations of patients consulting the nurse rather than the physician;
- the identification of aspects of patient care in general practice which may be undertaken by a nurse and to contrast those with ones requiring medical skill;
- and, the study of a sample of patients encouraged to take greater responsibility for their own health.

As of 1986, the results of such an evaluation were not available. The report on the interview with the nurse practitioner that is presented below must though be interpreted in this broader context.

The nurse practitioner was one member of the practice comprising three GPs and a receptionist, together with attached Health Authority community nurses including a community midwife, health visitor, and district nurse. The practice was run from a private house, not a health centre as in the previous case study. But it resembles the health centre in that patients were encouraged to drop in for a chat over coffee, children's paintings adorned the walls, and a small library had been set up, especially for younger children. Funding for the post was initially as part of the FPC remuneration scheme; once the evaluation project began, the NP's salary was paid for by the University of Birmingham.

A code of practice had to be drawn up prior to the establishment of the NP project. It is reproduced in Table 11.1. This was acceptable to the Medical Defence Union and the Royal College of Nursing, who both agreed to provide insurance cover.

One area where the nurse practitioner played a major role was that of diagnosing and treating simple illnesses as well as providing counselling on preventive and educative aspects of health care. Bowling (1981) in a study of delegation in general practice found that 62% of the sampled doctors stated that they had insufficient time to devote to patients whom they felt really need their attention. The major problem was that people consulted GPs over health matters which the GPs either defined as

Table 11.1: Supervision and Practice of the Nurse
Practitioner Research Project

1 The Nurse Practitioner (NP) will be supervised
  by a medical practitioner in the practice in
  which she is working, and by member of staff of
  the General Practice Teaching and Research Unit
  of the University of Birmingham.
2 The two medical supervisors will regularly
  assess the NP's competence to practise in this
  research project.
3 The NP will be consulted by patients only
  when a medical practitioner is on the surgery
  premises.
4 The NP will be competent (after appropriate
  additional training) to identify physical
  symptoms and signs which require medical
  attention and treatment.
5 There will be a system of referral within
  the general practice to allow immediate medical
  attention for any patient deemed by the NP to
  warrant it and there will be a list of
  conditions, sign/symptom combinations for which
  referral to the doctor is mandatory.
6 The NP's consultations will emphasise health
  education and the use of simple medication to
  encourage patients' self-reliance in the
  treatment of minor disorders.
7 The NP will not make first home visits. She
  may visit a patient only after the medical
  practitioner's initial assessment.
8 A patient may choose whom he wishes to
  consult, but if he consults the NP more than
  twice about the same illness, the NP must
  ensure that the patient is then seen by a
  medical practitioner.
9 The NP will record the presenting symptoms and
  her findings on examination, as well as any
  treatment recommended, in the medical notes.
  These will be available for her supervising
  general practitioner to read, at the end of
  each of the NP's consultations.

trivial in nature or as not really requiring their specific skills.

'It is one way of primary health care tackling social problems such as old age, and unemployment, for people who don't have anyone else to turn to. One GP at the surgery said to me the other day, "honestly, some mornings I feel just like a social worker", which was reflecting his own feelings really about having to deal with these sorts of problems. So maybe we do have to think again about primary health care' (NP).

Bowling (1981) found that nurses and GPs expressed reservations about the concept of initial screening by a non-physician. 51% of doctors and 32% of nurses felt that only qualified doctors could safely diagnose. Further, 32% of nurses stated that it was not within their role to screen patients, commenting, 'I wouldn't want to be a mini-doctor'. Finally, 37% of nurses and 28% of doctors felt that the patients would find such a development unacceptable: 'I think that there would be a punch up out there in the waiting room if anyone said that they weren't ill enough to see the doctor', a nurse commented. However, given the apprenticeship training with the GP on areas such as physical examinations, use of drugs, and advanced practice nursing, such a concern may be overstated. The nurse practitioner, rather than aiming to become a 'mini-doctor', argued that she offered a service different but complementary to that of the GPs.

'I see the whole approach as being fundamentally different really, the basic difference between a medical approach and a nursing approach. Something a NP from the United States said, I feel really sums it all up. She worked with a doctor, and he said, "look at what I do it's very similar to what you do". And she said, "yes, there is a lot of nursing in your consultations," and that's right, medicine is so formally structured'.

As for patient acceptability of screening by a non-physician, the way in which screening operated in the NP's surgery was that the patients chose which health worker they consulted:

'I am just in the surgery, and there is a notice which says, "We have a Nurse Practitioner working in the surgery and if you would like to see her just tell the receptionist. She has special training in the management of simple illnesses and many family health problems"'.

Patients appeared to readily consult the NP. They seemed to be very good at self selection, consulting the NP for simple health problems or over problems which required more of a counselling role.

INTERVIEWER: 'Did you find that patients consulted you easily in the beginning?'

NP: 'Yes amazingly, but it is the sort of practice where word gets around really quickly .... You know that people often feel very frightened of doctors, and in the States it has been found that if the NP says, " well I think that you should see the doctor", then they feel that they have been given an entree to the doctor, a kind of justification for being there. I often get that, "well I just wondered if it was worth bothering the doctor with" and that if I say " yes, that is a good idea", it provided an important justification for going'.

The nurse practitioner also found that women, especially younger women, consulted her very readily and in greater percentages than was average for the practice. In fact 73% of her patients were women. Although it is difficult to draw conclusions from this without further data, it is possible that for some sections of the population the NP was the health worker providing primary care as they would not consult a GP so readily. The possible intervening role of the receptionist cannot be ignored in recommending consultation with the NP if she felt the patients had little wrong with them.

The NP thus adopted an educative and preventive model of providing care based on an holistic assessment of the individual's needs. If a patient presented the NP with, for example, headaches, the NP stated that she immediately considered medical conditions such as a brain tumour or nephritis, or that this person may be under stress or have problems related to their social or economic circumstances.

> 'It is very much a whole person assessment which does include a physical assessment; and then based on what I find I refer to an appropriate agency. So if it's something physical and complex it's usually the GP, if it's simple I deal with it, and say "come back in three days", which is what the doctor would do anyway. So there is an overlap there. Or I can find that they really do have a problem and aren't coping at all well'.

How then does the NP respond to health problems which are linked to social and environmental problems? At the first level she sees her role as:

> 'helping them to cope. So if it's more of a social need, helping them to sort out who they should go to; ... or if it's counselling then I would offer first contact counselling. If it's a very long or complex problem like a marriage, then I would refer on to another counsellor, stating that I am always there for them to come back to'.

The NP in such consultations does not operate with a directive model of care, 'such as you must take things easier because I say it will be good for you', but instead has consciously adopted an approach of encouraging the client's self awareness of his/her own health. By building up a relationship of trust,

> 'the NP can become aware with the client of his/her own health needs and can allow the patient to set his/her own goals for improving their health. The client is thus not to be a passive accepting patient but becomes an assertive client, allowed and encouraged to ask questions, to disagree and to refuse'.

The NP argued that such an approach was important because,

> 'research shows that equipping patients to look after themselves more effectively will in the long run alter morbidity patterns'.

The practical application of such a philosophy involved the NP in consultations of at least twenty minutes in length in contrast to the five minute appointments of GPs. This includes the initial analysis of why the individual has presented and an evaluation of symptoms. Combined with this the NP also raised issues such as smoking or weight, in a manner which was likely to develop dialogue over health issues. The NP also offered to perform 'well person' check ups which provided another avenue into raising educative and preventive health issues.

Such an approach is not unproblematic to adopt for the nurse or client.

'Initially this sort of relationship is frightening for both nurse and client; after all it is comforting to be ordered to do something - "it is good for you" - and some patients will try and manipulate the NP into this style of education; for example "so you're telling me I should stop smoking then"'.

The nurse practitioner found that to begin with patients often sought to consult with her in the same way as they did with a doctor. Change was often very gradual:

'at first they did want to see me a bit in the same light of, "take this magic three times a day and you will be better", but once they saw that what I offered was different they pre-ferred it for some things'.

By adopting such a role the NP argued that she was addressing a very real need in the practice which had not been approached before.

In a survey of patient attitudes towards the NP that was conducted at the surgery, the NP and GPs found that several dominant reasons were given by patients for consulting her: 'she has time to talk with us'; and 'she understands, advises and helps'. As the NP stated,

'I think because societal structures are not the same in this area any more, families have moved .... For a lot of people, especially young women, I become an older sister or mother sort of role, they just see me as Barbara, they don't have to call me doctor or anything. So I think that we are fulfilling a very real need, and this may be something that we need to pay attention to in inner city practices'.

Through the adoption of such an 'educative, preventive and coping' model of health, the NP's treatment of simple illnesses changed with consequences for drug prescription. It must be remembered that it is illegal for a nurse to prescribe drugs, or to sign prescriptions; only a doctor is authorised to do so. With regard to the administration of medication,

'What we have done is to work out a code of practice. What I do is if say I have a child with a middle ear infection, I know the signs and symptoms which I group together, and when I have satisfied these criteria myself I go to the GP and say "I have found this and this antibiotic is what I would prescribe" and I write out the prescription and the GP then either says "OK that's fine" and signs it, or he says "no I think I had better have a look". So in effect I write the prescription and the doctor signs it. Now that may sound outrageous, but if you put it in the context of people phoning up and saying "can I have an antibiotic as I am ill?" and then the receptionist writes it out, I mean we all know that happens in general practice a lot, so what I do doesn't sound so bad. Indeed, patients come to our receptionist and say that, but she says "well you need to see someone"'.

Section 6 of the NP's code of practice (see Table 11.1) states:

'the NP's consultations will emphasise health education and the use of simple medication to encourage patients' self-reliance in the treatment of minor disorders'.

The NP found that adhering to this code combined with her 'coping' model of health both worked to actively reduce the amount of drugs given to patients. As she states:

'In the three years that I have been in the practice, I have given a total of 14% of my patients prescriptions, and it is even less now because the patients are realising that I am not a soft touch, as I go into all other sorts of coping, believing that it is far better to avoid drugs whereever possible'.

As a final comment, the nurse practitioner identified differences between herself and a practice nurse.

'I am autonomous and able to find my own depth, which is slightly unusual. I don't wear a uniform, so I am seen as a practitioner rather than a nurse who does all the practical things. Also, if say a patient comes in feeling dizzy and I think that some blood tests are required, then I just set them up and don't have to ask the GP about them. So in that sense I am more autonomous, as I can think of what needs to be done, do it, and bring a patient back for review. I also do a lot of teaching in my session'.

Her autonomy was restricted only to the extent of the code of practice established for the project. Consultation with the GP was readily available, but referral was only made when the nurse practitioner felt that the patient's conditions deemed it necessary.

THE EAST END OF LONDON PROJECT

The interview with the nurse practitioner in the Birmingham project has highlighted the potential of a nurse with extended training to act in a diagnostic manner, to treat and prescribe drugs under medical supervision, to screen patients, and to develop a relationship with the patient allowing both an exploration of the underlying nature of their health problem (its broader social basis) and counselling and health promotion. She was however not the only nurse practitioner explicitly with that title within the British NHS. There was also the case of Sister Barbara Burke-Masters, working in the East End of London, since 1980.
Her clientele was untypical and of little attraction to GPs, consisting of down-and-outs, tramps and vagrant alcoholics - homeless persons who found it difficult to obtain acceptance onto a GP's list. She acted as an 'autonomous' practitioner, both in counselling, and treating and prescribing drugs to her patients. While in the

Birmingham project, the prescriptions had to be signed by a GP, Burke-Master's supervisor prescribed a range of about 12 drugs in bulk to her (antibiotics, tranquillisers and pain killers) (Cohen, 1984). She decided what to dispense, after taking the patient's history and so on, and tried to give health educative advice. She was also autonomous in her working conditions, being apart from the supervising GP's practice. Her 'surgery' was contained within a 'bare dimly-lit room .... The main furniture is just the desk, two chairs and a large cupboard containing her drugs and equipment' (p.22).

The funding for her post - a half time position at Nurse Sister level - was initially provided by the St George's Men's Care Unit Charity but the local Tower Hamlets Health Authority subsequently paid her salary indirectly in recognition of the contribution she was making to primary care. Nevertheless the Health Authority could not officially recognise Burke-Master's work, and the District Nursing Officer admitted to misgivings about her rather 'idiosyncratic' approach (Gaze, 1985, p.20). This unease was shared by some voluntary agencies who regarded a nurse practitioner as the harbinger of segregated, second class care for homeless people, and by many GPs and hospital consultants (in constrast to the medical support in the Birmingham NP project). In late 1984 the management committee of the Charity issued an ultimatum that she should obtain proper authorisation to carry on or the premises would be closed. Before that could happen officers from the Pharmaceutical Society inspected her surgery in 1985 and confiscated the restricted drugs which she dispensed. This action effectively ended Burke-Master's four-and-a-half years work with the homeless. She has received considerable support from one local GP, and some encouragement from a few consultants who accepted referrals, but the overwhelming impression is of a climate of suspicion and antagonism despite the fact that 'she had been providing a needed service and one which the NHS accepted while refusing to recognise' (p.20).

NURSES IN GENERAL PRACTICE

The interview with the Birmingham NP and the brief account of the East London project highlight the potential of an extended role for the nurse in primary care, in terms of providing a type of service which most GPs find little time for (prevention and counselling) or serving a group currently receiving no or little care. Other examples of innovation in PHC may be documented. There is the case of a community psychiatric nurse, working from a North London group practice who is undertaking 'preventive psychiatry', providing counselling and behaviour therapy. Such a person elsewhere tends to be based in the hospital context. This experiment the GPs describe in glowing terms:

> 'He must have paid for himself several times over in cuts in prescribing and hospital referrals ... (He) has changed the character of the practice' (Feinmann, 1985, p.1229).

The post is funded by the local Health Authority. There is too the example of the nurse practitioners in the health centre described in Chapter Ten, both of whom have areas of special responsibility (for screening and the elderly).

Looking more broadly, there is an array of nurses working in general practice. Not only are there nurse practitioners, but also 'practice nurses' who undertake a supportive role to the GP in relation to patient treatment and are increasingly adopting a health promotion function (Bowling, 1981; Sanders et al, 1986). These nurses are employed under the FPC renumeration scheme. There is also a range of nurses employed by the local Health Authority, within the category of community nursing. There are 'community midwives' providing care and support to the newborn baby and mother until handing over to the 'health visitor' once the baby reaches ten days old. The health visitor performs a preventive function - monitoring the child's development, giving advice to the mother on the care of the child, and referring where necessary to the GP. In addition, she has a comparable role in relation to the elderly. There is also the 'district nurse' who provides a treatment and caring service, for example, to the elderly in bathing, or for the newly discharged (changing dressings), or looking after the housebound. All three tend to be attached to a GP's practice, although in the past they were geographically zoned. Finally, there are 'family planning nurses', 'school nurses' and so on.

Not only is it apparent that there are potentially large numbers of nurses working outside of the hospital, be they attached to a GP, directly employed by a GP, or based in the hospital, but also they perform a wide range of tasks. In addition, these nurses are in varying degrees subject to medical supervision - for example, the practice nurse within the surgery compared to the health visitor or midwife on a home visit. There is the possibility of an overlap in their roles and responsibilities and even a potential confusion over who is doing what.

An OPCS survey (Dunnell and Dobbs, 1982) sheds some light on the activities and potential role overlap of nurses working in the community. Looking firstly at the practice nurse employed by the GP, 60% of her time was spent in clinics, 36% in schools hospitals or elsewhere, and only 4% on home visits. In terms of tasks carried out, 34% of the time was spent undertaking tests, assessments, screening or other technical procedures; 7% in giving advice or counselling; and 58% on non-clinical activities. This comprised clerical and administrative duties relating to her job as a nurse (26%), reception duty (16%) and telephone calls, meetings and so on (16%). In contrast, both the health visitor and the district nurse spent much of their time on home visits (56% and 89% respectively) and less in the clinics (26% and 5% respectively). The health visitor had a large amount of non-clinical duties (55% of her time) but also undertook advice and counselling work (33%). Her non-clinical activities involved clerical and administrative work (30%) and telephone calls, meetings, teaching and so on (25%). The district nurse's time was mostly spent in technical nursing care (52%), with 11% on advice and counselling and 35% in non-clinical activities. This non-clinical work covered clerical and administrative tasks (19%) and telephone calls, teaching and so on (16%).

One point of difference between the nurses employed by and those attached to GPs is worthy of note. For the latter, it is the District Health Authority who is their employer, and it is to that organisation that the nurse looks for managerial accountability. Such nurses are essentially independent of immediate medical supervision, working as autonomous practitioners, perhaps resulting in a relatively high satisfaction of community nursing staff. Their working relationships with the GPs depend to a large extent on personalities and individual predilection. In contrast,the practice nurse is most often directly employed by the GP, who fixes both her conditions of service, including pay, and job responsibilities. Considerable variety is therefore likely. As for pay, the GP is reimbursed up to 70% of the cost, subject generally to the maximum Whitley Council level for a Sister grade. The GP can decide to pay above such a level, but any excess has to be met by the practice and not the FPC.

Hart (1985a) has recently drawn to the attention of fellow GPs the possibility and benefit of employing practice nurses, pointing out that

'... another 27,000 skilled workers (could be added) to our present overworked teams, and as matters now stand neither the Treasury nor the DHSS could stop it' (p.1163).

One potential means for improving primary health care and general practice in particular, would be for GPs to employ a practice nurse especially if the nurse is given responsibility for preventive and educative aspects of health care. A mere increase in numbers is not sufficient, but rather a change in attitude is required, moving away from the methods of training and rewarding GPs,

'... which perpetuate one man bands when we need orchestras .... In particular, we need to think about new definitions of what constitutes a good doctor and a good nurse working outside hospital' (Hart, 1985b, p.29).

The Cumberlege Report (DHSS, 1986a) advocated a discontinuation of the reimbursement scheme for nurses, but this was rejected by the Secretary of State (DHSS, 1986b). Furthermore, it argued for nurses in general practice to be under the supervision of a Neighbourhood Community Nurse Manager.

TOWARDS A GENERIC COMMUNITY NURSE?

The debate about general practice, its quality and the workers involved has gained fresh impetus with the publication of two important discussion papers (DHSS, 1986a and b). Cumberlege (DHSS, 1986a) argues for the potential of the nurse practitioner role in the 'new' PHC world, but medical opinion is unconvinced. Stilwell has pointed to the NP's role as being to complement the GP's role with nursing skills. This would recognise the value of the nursing model in primary care and the necessity of team working or collaborative practice.

Fears of GPs over the threat of an extended role for the nurse may be exaggerated. The NP comments:

'I don't think it will bring down the GP's status.... (They) are often rather miffed at their image as the generalist, and get frowned upon by hospital consultants. If there is another first line of contact (it may) improve their status'.

In addition, the GPs in the Birmingham practice were attracted by the prospect of a two-way dialogue. Knowing there was someone in the practice to whom they could refer a patient for discussion over diet, weight, and general counselling or for screening and monitoring of blood pressure was seen as very valuable. Furthermore, the incorporation of nursing skills and expertise may help extend preventive activities, including the appreciation of environmentally related illnesses and stress.

The two nurse practitioners discussed here represent only a tiny proportion of nurses working in general practice. Indeed, some practice nurses appear to undertake a not dissimilar range of activities (see Chapter 10 and Sanders et al, 1986), even if their attitudes and predominant nursing orientation may differ, with the practice nurse seeing her job in the context of 'helping the doctor with his patients' and the attached nurse in terms of 'the patient needs (our) care' (Reedy, 1980). Traditional nursing tasks (such as dressings and injections), added to areas such as examining ears, monitoring blood pressure and hearts (ECGs), need extension, as Stilwell argues, to areas of counselling, teaching and promoting health. It is thus an 'extension' to the nurse's lexicon,not the development of a 'new' type of worker in PHC, that is seemingly being advocated.

The reasons why a nurse should wish to work in general practice, employed by a GP, are not straightforward. Hart (1985b) draws attention to the likely job conditions: lack of a pension scheme, no or little organised in-service training, no career structure, and perhaps no written contract. But hours are flexible, as too are job definitions; autonomy in the work exists and there is opportunity to work within a team where to some extent clinical information and decisions are shared (p.29). Stilwell no doubt would add, on the positive side, the opportunity to apply the unique skills of nursing to PHC.

In terms of cost effectiveness, extended training for a practice nurse (or nurse practitioner) must be perceived as viable (Bowling, 1985b). But training in what and for what role is a matter of some debate. Turton (1985) points out that

> 'separate training for different community nurses is expensive. More important, it may not be the best preparation to meet communities' health needs or promote effective teamwork' (p.25).

Moreover, it is argued that a generic 'public health' or 'primary care nurse' is required (Kratz, 1985). The lack of training opportunities for practice nurses has also not gone unnoticed. A RCN Working Party (RCN, 1984) suggested some form of organised training for them.

In the context of the independent contractor status of the GP, whether the potential of an extended role of a nurse in general practice will be fulfilled is an open question. Hart (1985a and b) points to attitudes as being critical. It is interesting to note Stilwell's comments early on in the nurse practitioner project:

> 'The project is not only about a nurse practitioner in England, it is also making vulnerable the nursing role in order to expose its intrinsic value and its uniqueness among health workers. It is a project about nurses and doctors dropping their traditional guards and sharing their knowledge with each other and with their patients' (Stilwell, 1982a, p.1803).

This needs to be juxtaposed with Hart's comments:

> 'current conventional wisdom seems to be that doctors and nurses will move further apart, as independent and increasingly autonomous practitioners' (Hart, 1985b, p.29).

Expanded Role for the Nurse or New Worker?

The issue of professionalism and teamwork are brought to the forefront of attention.

'Real progress in general practice depends on a restructuring of primary care, to increase both public investment and public accountability'(ibid).

Whether the Green Paper on primary care (DHSS, 1986b) and the Cumberlege Report (DHSS, 1986a) will lead to a move in the requisite direction remains to be seen. The case of the nurse practitioner is one of a call for dialogue between health workers, not for a tightening and demarcation of professional rights and controls in general practice. Such conflicts invariably exclude the patient's interests. In the words of the nurse practitioner:

'What we do need to look at is what patients want and need .... We are very good at looking at what everyone else wants, but the poor old patient doesn't even get asked'.

Chapter 12

THE EVALUATION OF HEALTH MANPOWER PRACTICES

In this final Chapter, discussion turns to the evaluation of existing manpower policies and practices. An emphasis on evaluation has been a noticeable feature of recent managerial initiatives in the health services, and it is necessary to begin by exploring the particular interpretation adopted in official (i.e. DHSS) accounts. The significance accorded to evaluation will then be set against how it is applied in Health Authorities. This confirms that evaluation is far from being the straight-forward technical exercise that the rationalist NHS planning system portrays, thus directing attention to the political nature and context of the health manpower process. This perspective is too often absent in 'official accounts' of evaluation, and in consequence has led to a misrepresentation of the conditions which alternatively encourage inertia, innovation, conflict and co-operation. A major segment of this Chapter is therefore taken up with a more extensive view of what health manpower evaluation might comprise. This is especially important in analysing the case studies presented in the previous three Chapters in order to consider the possibilities for the diffusion of manpower practices consonant with the development of primary health care.

THE FOCUS ON EVALUATION

Assessment of the present state of the NHS has been a long running saga, not that this has provided too much common ground for those evaluating the performance of the health services. The Royal Commission on the National Health Service Report (1979) is instructive. This bears witness to the problems involved in specifying the aims of the NHS, how these are to be measured, and the interpretation to be placed on such evaluation. In a magisterial analysis of performance evaluation in the health services, Klein (1982) suggests that this is necessarily problematic because health care is distinguished 'by its complexity, heterogeneity, uncertainty and ambiguity' (p. 386). The discussion in earlier Chapters has illustrated these aspects in terms of health manpower. The 'complexity' is demonstrated in the diverse skills represented in the NHS workforce, and reinforced by its size and distribution across the country. The 'heterogeneity' is evident in the comparable breadth of services provided from acute care hospitals to those in the community. 'Uncertainty' points to the difficulty in establishing a precise, causal connection between inputs and outputs: what, for example, is the relative impact of nursing and occupational therapy for the mentally handicapped? As the Royal Commission Report (1979) demonstrated, if a high doctor-to-population ratio is so widely commended, then why is it associated with 'a relatively high perinatal mortality rate' (para. 3.19)? Finally, much of the information on the health services demonstrates high levels of 'ambiguity'. Is an increase in patients treated by the NHS an indicator of its success in providing care, or of its failure to prevent illness?

If these aspects of health care inhibit performance evaluation, the task is further constrained by its organisational context. The NHS is asked to:

'square two circles. First it is an attempt to reconcile central government responsibility for the financing of the service with delegation of responsibility for service delivery to peripheral authorities. Second, it is an attempt to combine the doctrine of public accountability with the doctrine of professional autonomy' (Klein, 1982, p. 387).

Hence the story of evaluation in the NHS has unfolded against a backcloth of conflict between central and local Authorities, as well as Health Authorities and Health Departments, and the health professions (mainly medicine).

The early years of the NHS were characterised by a number of attempts to rationalise the organisation and delivery of the health services, but little headway, or even inclination, was demonstrated towards stricter evaluation procedures, especially in the field of health manpower. A number of inquiries were conducted into various staff groups and these suggested that the professional providers of health care - especially doctors - were the pre-eminent arbiters of manpower issues. A harbinger of more recent thinking was however contained in the Guillebaud Report (1956) which examined how far the NHS was efficient, and gave value for money. It emphasised the comparative performance of Health Authorities, as advocated by the Ministry of Health, in order to determine their league position on such indicators as 'average occupancy of beds, length of stay of patients, bed turnover, turnover interval, waiting time etc.' (p.131). Klein (1982, p. 389) makes the point that the Guillebaud Committee was convinced that improved information was crucial but their focus was slanted towards the 'efficiency' rather than the 'effectiveness' of services provided to patients.

Through the 1960s pressure mounted, emanating from the Treasury in particular, to ensure that central government departments provided detailed medium and long term forecasts of their activities and costs. An increasingly favoured exemplar was the management structures and styles associated with large scale, private industry. The aim was to refurbish the NHS on the basis of a structural re-organisation allied with the introduction of a revamped managerial ethos. In this unitary model, any lingering thoughts of a 'blue-print' goal for the health service were displaced by a concern with improving the 'rationality' of decision making. The criteria for assessing the merits of the NHS shifted from a rather vague notion of the 'public interest' - typically left to the medical profession to interpret - to the 'new' planning goals.

The rational model gave prominence to the significance of evaluating performance and ensuring accountability of lower to higher level tiers. The 'Grey Book' (DHSS, 1972) details the ways in which 'progress according to plan', 'to agreed objectives, targets and budgets', and 'efficiency and economy' are at the forefront of management thinking. In broad terms, the official concern has been to produce a 'better' performance through:

. objective setting and identification of
  problems;
. formulation of policies to achieve
  objectives; and
. implementation and monitoring of policies.

The contrast is with the context for health planning
it replaced, which, insofar as it existed,
emphasised broad objectives, such as a hospital
building programme. The new system focussed
typically on a detailed and explicit scheme for the
formulation and implementation of policies. This
altered the standards by which a plan/policy was
judged as 'good' or not, and gave prominence to
central priorities.
    Official accounts categorise the whole planning
exercise as a 'learning process'. One important
aspect of this education of local Health Authorities
and health care practitioners was that evaluation
was a mechanism for improved central control.
Underpinning the official discourse was 'the
dominance of the centre and the weakness of the
learning mode' (Glennerster, 1981, p. 43). A
determined effort was mounted to counter the
perceived 'failures' in policy making and 'poor'
performance. It is significant that the DHSS
attempted to achieve this not through direct
intervention in local autonomy in service provision,
but instead through a steady flow of guidelines -
such as manpower targets, priority services, and
funding levels. This concentrated attention on
whether Authorities were achieving centrally agreed
objectives without raising questions about the
intelligence on which those aims were based. It
spotlighted the NHS's own view of its organisational
effectiveness to the exclusion of 'outside'
evaluation (Klein, 1982, pp. 398-9).
    Hence, while the DHSS was publicly voicing its
ambition to delegate authority downwards to the
appropriate level, it was by other means enhancing
its control through monitoring and review - what
Hill (1979) has referred to as 'post-hoc'
evaluation. Other evaluation techniques, such as
randomised controlled trials, cost benefit, and
cost-effectiveness analysis, have been generally
encouraged because they link with the general aim
to make the NHS more cost conscious and efficient,
but they do not occupy the same pre-eminent position
as monitoring and review.
    A further aspect of evaluation, or an issue
which runs parallel to it, is that of
implementation. If one of the major stimulants

behind evaluation in the NHS planning system has been the pressure to contain costs, a further potent factor has been policy 'shortfall', or the realisation that plan formulation and policy implementation do not follow each other unproblematically. The factors underlying any such 'implementation gap' have been the subject of considerable debate, and very contrasting perspectives have been offered (Harrison, 1985). Within the planning model adopted by the NHS any shortcomings are cast primarily as a failure to keep local Health Authorities in step with central preferences. The problem is categorised by Majone and Wildavsky (1979) as 'implementation-as-control'. This accords with a basic premise of the rational model introduced in the 1970s that mechanisms had to be found for integrating lower tier plans with central priorities and resource strategies.

Insofar as the analysis of implementation involves an appreciation that 'programmes have to be brought to life' (WHO, 1981, p. 7), it confronts some of the assumptions built into the unitary model about the character of the decision making process, and specifically about the applicability of a top-down approach to the NHS context. According to Hunter (1983), research

> 'challenges, first, the assumption that policy-making and implementation are quite separate activities and, second, the assumption that they conform, to a top-down (i.e. hierarchical) managerial model in which policy is handed down from above to be implemented by front-line operators' (p. 135).

While the central Health Departments may always travel in hope, they are not so naive as to suppose that the NHS will instantly jump when higher level 'orders' are issued. Nor have central Health Departments the ambition to regulate the day-to-day activities of Health Authorities across the country. It is nevertheless intended that in broad terms the evaluation mechanisms will provide a direct and indirect encouragement (or constraint) to reduce policy 'failures'. This ambition brings Health Authorities generally into frequent conflict with the professionals providing the health services.

The medical profession is widely regarded as a group that displays a high level of occupational control, both in its dealings with its clients and the NHS as its 'employer'. Considerable effort is invested in maintaining this privileged position, and there is ample evidence of struggles on the part of other occupational groups to 'usurp' some of that dominance and control over their own destiny for themselves (Larkin, 1983; Dingwall and McIntosh, 1978). Professional groups, and the strategies and tactics they adopt therefore are important elements in the form of evaluation employed in the NHS. Hitherto, it has been commonplace to regard the medical profession as dominant in the organisation and delivery of services to patients. The presumption has been that its control over health care encompasses a considerable power over its own, and even other, manpower.

While some detect a decline in such 'medical hegemony' (Armstrong, 1976), others are more convinced that the challenging interests have not completely won the day. Alford (1975), for example, portrays the main conflict in the health services as between the 'professional monopolists' and the 'corporate rationalisers'. These latter have grown in number with the increased size, complexity and bureaucratisation of the health services. They include a wide range of management and administrative staff, from general managers through to more specialised manpower planners and personnel officers. Much of the recent policy debate in the NHS has been cast as a developing challenge by this group to the professional monopolists, and in particular the medical profession (Mercer and Long, 1981; Ham, 1981). The corporate rationalisers have been pressing for a framework for health care evaluation which is not determined by the producer groups.

Yet if Alford's schema is a useful backcloth to recent manpower debates, there are grounds for regarding it as too polarised. There are in practice manifest conflicts both within and between the several interests in the health services which must be recognised in order to understand the detail of health manpower. For example, the monolithic front of the medical profession hides many internal interest groups and fragile alliances. Similarly, Alford has difficulty in accounting for the competitive strategies employed against the medical profession, by other professionals such as nurses and physiotherapists. For the latter groups, their input is rather more to extend their own occupational control (vis-a-vis both medicine and the corporate rationalisers) than to protect an entrenched power base. What is at issue is whether the considerable clinical autonomy that professionals still enjoy extends to the health manpower process. It has been documented (Haywood and Alaszewski, 1980; Haywood and Hunter, 1982; Hunter, 1983) how the routines and practices adopted by those in front-line positions effectively become public policy in a reversal of the top-down model. It is unlikely that manpower policies are so different, although it is possible that more stringent monitoring and control of manpower has begun to make inroads into this aspect of professional discretion.

Evaluation of the health manpower process has then more sides to it than is implied by a straightforward preparation of a balance sheet to determine 'success' or 'failure'. The unitary model of a rationally ordered organisation provides the official yardstick of actual practice. The discussion which follows attempts to pursue the merits of this model for understanding the health manpower process in general, while also searching for clues about the conditions and strategies which appear to encourage the development of primary health care.

EVALUATING MANPOWER PRACTICE

Without any monitoring (a 'soft' version of evaluation), how do the policy makers and budget holders know if the organisation is on target? A 'harder' interpretation of evaluation suggests an assessment of the extent to which explicit objectives have been achieved, searching out reasons why not, and, for the exercise to have anything more than a symbolic or negative sanctioning role, also indicating how the objectives can be reached given the organisation's present position. More prosaically, two main approaches are pursued here: firstly, to identify the evaluative schema used in the context of health manpower; and secondly, to develop and employ an evaluative checklist based on a view of 'what ought to be' or 'what could be'.

Within the present study an attempt was made to glean from the Regional and the central Health Departments' manpower planners (that is, among those tiers with the main responsibility for monitoring) the criteria that they intended to employ for their review of manpower within the 1985/6 strategic planning round. A short questionnaire was circulated (in April 1985) asking:

'how the manpower element in the District plan was being evaluated . . . the criteria and any associated methodology? . . . (and) to what extent is emphasis placed on the quantitative side of manpower demand and supply, and also on the qualitative issues of role, substitution and productivity?'

Three main features emerged in the replies. Firstly, there was the major consideration of the affordability of the plan and its associated manpower; the District's plan must fit revenue targets. To this end, many Authorities had to complete SASP tables (Summary Analysis of Strategic Plans) indicating by care group the staffing numbers required, quantified for each of the ten years of the planning period, and subdivided by skill mix (qualified, unqualified, learners). In addition, the reviewers may apply 'average' staffing costs to check on the financial implications of the plan. As a sub-aspect of this criterion, adherence to projected manpower ceilings and revenue targets was assessed, particularly with respect to central guidance on direct patient versus non-patient related staff numbers and costs. A second factor involved the application of performance indicators to District plans, or at least adherence to Regional and/or DHSS guidance. For example, if a District currently had a low level of allied health professional staff in relation to such features as its population base and bed provision, and in the ten year plan it showed little evidence of expanding such staff, this would be queried. Or, if a District currently had a low level of such staff, compared to other Authorities in the Region, and its staffing projections indicated at the end of the planning period it would have the largest number of such staff in the Region, again this would be queried, to check whether the need existed, and to see if such growth could be achieved in practice. The third criterion was linked to the potential achievement of the supply of desired staff. A DHA's manpower strategy was thus examined on the potential success of its training and recruitment programme. In addition to these crucial manpower factors, other more general criteria are likely to have been utilised in order to review and monitor service developments and plans: for example, the explicit adherence of the strategy to central priorities, and the pursuit of desirable service provision (a question such as, 'is the District developing its services to meet at least the identified "minimum standard"?'). Further, within the District itself, additional manpower factors would be specified: for example, a 'case of need' to justify a new post, manpower requirements based on an assessment of workload, and not just professional judgement or norms, and keeping manpower within the target set.

However, while the above three criteria may be the major ones operating on the manpower side in the British NHS as regards strategic planning, one can queston whether these are a sufficient and wide ranging set of factors. Indeed, the very notion of the health manpower process expounded by Mejia (1978) and others, and used as the guiding structure for both the research and this text, suggests a more extensive list. It is a separate, and later, question as to why the NHS appears to pursue only the three factors noted above, and what the implications might be for health care planning and provision. Accordingly, Table 12.1 presents an attempt to draw out a more elaborate set of evaluative criteria founded upon the three dimensions of the health manpower process – planning, production and management. In addition, a fourth aspect is appended, involving the integration (or integrating mechanisms) of the three dimensions in order to achieve the desired health objectives.

Such a checklist involves, as does any evaluation, an implicit statement of what is deemed important by the evaluator. Evaluation, as is implementation, is thus explicitly a political activity, and prefaced on normative choices and judgements. Two points are worthy of note. Firstly, the evaluative questions, while implying an ideal for health manpower practices, are suggested as depicting one way of approaching the area. This explicitly pursues and addresses the link between manpower and service provision to the achievement of health objectives for the population. Secondly, attention lies not in adherence to the spirit of the approach but in an optimisation of each category and the health manpower process as a whole.

The issue of evaluation can be approached from another angle altogether, based in part on theory and in part on practice. That is, (un)desirable manpower practices or innovations, and/or (un)desirable features of manpower distribution and utilisaton, for example, can be examined. In this regard consideration may be given to issues such

Table 12.1: An Evaluative Checklist of the Health Manpower Process

	Planning	Production	Management	Integration
Objectives:	To specify the number of teams and their composition needed to improve the level of health up to a proposed level.	To produce x people of y type	To determine manpower distribution and productivity standards, patterns of utilisation and non-labour inputs.	To ensure that the planning, production, and management dimensions are integrated to achieve the health objectives.
Critical Questions:	To what extent is there a systematic assessment of manpower requirements based on: *an exploration of current and future roles in relation to the health objectives? *an examination of current and future skill mixes in relation to the health objectives? *a multi-disciplinary team approach orientated to the provision of the desired level of health? To what extent is there a systematic assessment of manpower supply based on: *an exploration of existing and future stocks of manpower? *an exploration of existing and future flows of manpower? To what extent are manpower requirements and supply 'matched'?	How far, and in what ways, are the education and training organisations and systems: *responsive to service needs? *orientated to service needs? How far, and in what ways, are the curricula linked to expected and desired manpower roles?	To what extent are persons with desirable characteristics recruited? To what extent is manpower utilised optimally? To what extent is manpower sufficiently motivated? To what extent is the quality of services maximised?	How far, and in what ways, are costs taken into account? How, and in what ways, are plans implemented? How is the implementation of the plan monitored?

as (over)specialisation, occupationally based (rather than multidisciplinary) team planning, role and skill changes and substitution. These issues can be explored at the level of theory:

. how are they to be defined?
. what might be their respective strengths and weaknesses in service delivery?
. what factors might encourage or inhibit their pursuit?

At the level of practice, a further range of questions is suggested:

. how are they defined and understood by the health practitioners, the policy makers and the consumers?
. are they, and in what ways, perceived as problematic in service delivery (in meeting health care needs)?
. what aspects, or which practices should be fostered and which should be discouraged?

Tables 12.2 to 12.5 present one set of perceptions at the level of theory in respect of specialisation, a multi-disciplinary team approach, role questioning/enlargement, and professionalism. These are presented only to exemplify the first stage in this evaluative perspective. The second, and critical phase, is to document such issues in the perceptions of health practitioners and consumers. Three perspectives on evaluating health manpower practices have been suggested here - identifying the practitioners' schema, employing an evaluative checklist based on the notion of the health manpower process, and critically reviewing aspects of manpower practice against views of practitioners and consumers to search out areas to foster or avoid. How the NHS reviews itself has already been identified, both in terms of explicit criteria used by Regional and central manpower planners and also implicitly in the discussions elsewhere in this text. As to how it fares under the examination of the evaluative checklist of Table 12.1, the following section will help to clarify, in identifying areas of emphasis, omission and possibilities for innovation.

APPLYING THE EVALUATIVE CHECKLIST

Looking at the NHS in the 1980s, the focal motif

Table 12.2:   Specialisation in Medicine

Definition
. 'A level of knowledge and skill in a particular aspect of medical work which is greater than that acquired during the course of basic medical education and internship.'
. 'A specialist is a doctor who has the knowledge, skills and experience judged necessary for the independent practice of a specific type of medical work.' (WHO, 1985c, p. 10)

Potential Strengths
. To maintain and improve the quality of practice. To provide genuine legal protection for the public.

Potential Weakenesses
. Narrow specialisation leads to repeated referral of the patient from expert to expert, entailing inconvenience, frustration and added costs (repetitive tests etc), discontinuity of care, and narrowing of clinical practice which together engender an 'anti-holistic' approach to medicine' (p. 13).
. Inflexibility of education and training, rigidity within and between specialties, effect on career choices, and (un)employment prospects.
. Questionable attempt to meet health needs.

Ways to Modify Effect with a View to Increasing Quality (Effectiveness, Efficiency and Acceptability of Care)
. Exploration and understanding of the health needs of the population, and the relationship of need and demand.
. Exploration of the contribution of the range of staff to health care (the notion of multi-disciplinary teamwork).
. Encouragement of role flexibility in professional education and training.

Long-Term Detrimental Effects
. Greater differences in standards of care, between those who can afford expensive services and those that cannot.
. Increase cost of health care (specialist manpower and associated costs).

. Effect on career choices and employment prospects.
. Opportunity costs - specialists preferring to practise in higher income (and attractive) areas, leading to a more inequitable distribution of health care.

Action Required
. To explore what specialists do.
. To identify if overspecialisation exists.
. To clarify negative and positive features in order to build on the latter.

Table 12.3: Multidisciplinary Teamwork Approach

Definition
. Exploration of the relative contribution each member of a team can make to patient care, where the team comprises a group of workers with requisite skills, set up with the specific task of providing a level of health care to a defined set of patients.

Potential Strengths
. Through teamwork, a holistic approach to care.
. Easy transfer of patient onto another team member, leading to continuity of care.
. Fostering a loosening of professional boundaries (and a challenge to them).
. Clarification of who does what.

Factors Actively Preventing such an Approach
. Professional rigidity.
. Requires trust and good working relationships which do not currently exist across professions.
. Physician wants to stay 'in control' as team leader, with consequences for the maintenance of traditional role definitions.

Table 12.4:   Role Questioning and Exploration

Definition
. Exploration and examination of the current
  role definition and performance of a health
  worker, in relation to the health care
  provided, with a view to defining and
  performing a more appropriate role.

Potential Strengths
. Clarification of role and responsibilities and
  the relevance to patient care.
. Encourages assessment of alternative manpower
  mixes to provide service.
. Fosters consideration of who is the most
  appropriate to undertake a particular task
  (role enlargement, and substitution).
. Encourages responsiveness in terms of staff
  (roles) to changing health needs.

Factors Actively Preventing Such An Approach
. Rigidity of training and education encourages
  adherence to traditional role patterns, and
  relationships.
. Maintenance of existing professional
  boundaries, and specialisations.

Factors to Encourage
. Discussion across professional boundaries.
. Joint education and training across health
  workers.
. Experimentation with 'new' types of workers
  (e.g. nurse practitioner).

Table 12.5: Professionalism

Definition
. A profession 'is an occupational group whose
  members all have a specific formal education of
  considerable duration and that formal training
  is geared towards the specific occupation; so,
  a profession implies a monopoly' (Hofoss, 1986,
  p. 202).
. 'Professionalisation' - the process and
  circumstances under which people in an
  occupation attempt to turn it into a profession
  (control over knowledge, and its application
  and formal training).
. 'Professionalism' - acting in pursuit or
  protection of one's profession's (professional)
  self interest.

Potential Strengths
. High, and independently set, and accepted
  (publicly) standards of care.
. Builds on patients' expectations.
. Professions exist, and changes to health
  services can be discussed with them.

Potential Weaknesses
. Over-rigidity in role - demarcation of who does
  what, leading to problems if a 'critical' staff
  member cannot be recruited.
. Encourages specialisation.
. Implies primacy of medical knowledge carrying
  over to non-medical aspects of health care.

Ways to Modify Effect with a View to Increasing
Quality of Care
. Incentives to multi-disciplinary teamwork.
. Changes in legal responsibilities.
. Joint training and education with other health
  workers.

is the examination of the management dimension. The development of performance indicators, the introduction of general management, and the Annual Review Process are examples of the depth of interest. Cost containment and managerial efficiency are the catchphrases. In more particular manpower terms, manpower targets and vacancy review systems are two instances of criteria to 'manage' and 'control' manpower (costs). The response within the professions has been to draw up 'cases of need'. As the postal questionnaire data show, professional judgement as a basis for estimating manpower requirements is no longer acceptable. Resort has to be made to activity, and in some cases to quality (for example, Criteria for Care and Monitor in nursing forecasts).

It is interesting to note that while in nursing attention to dependency and other workload approaches has a long history, original interest in the area arose in the context of the planning dimension of the health manpower process, that is, to assist in determining how many staff were required. A shift in location is occurring, the methods being used to both justify existing (and any future) numbers and explore utilisation. Clinicians and allied health professionals have also started to move towards a workload based approach. Norms, drawn up on the basis of peers' professional judgement, or the use of professional judgement by senior and experienced staff run counter to the planning culture within the NHS.

Accordingly, management concern with manpower utilisation, in order to control costs and to live within tightly constraining financial limits, predominates with little apparent attention, except at the margin, to service quality and the achievement of desired health objectives. Efficiency, to the detriment of effectiveness and acceptability, is the thrust. In terms of the checklist, while the motivation of staff and the exploration of the quality of services are given a token priority, little attempt is made to optimise their achievement. Manpower utilisation, in a context of restrained budgets, has to be the overriding aim, with inevitable consequences for staff morale and the quality of service provision.

Turning to the production dimension, as the analysis of the different professions has shown (Chapters 4-6, and 8), this aspect is in essence perceived by NHS officers as too many steps removed to either influence or have control over. Indeed, it is seen as the responsibility of someone else, 'higher up' the organisation, be it Region, DHSS, or NHS Management Board. As the discussion in Chapter 3 pointed out, the production sector is outside or largely independent of the Districts, or even the NHS. Curriculum content tends to be professionally controlled and influenced mostly by tradition. Indeed, changes in the context of education and training have arisen not from pressures applied to the profession, but from internally generated ones. Project 2000 (UKCC, 1986) is a case in point. Also, two year (part time) vocational training schemes have been established for GPs and more recently for GDPs, as final preparation for their role in primary care, after six or so years of medical or dental education. The professions themselves have argued for such moves, not least to enhance professional status. But the root cause lies in the character of medical/dental education, and its apparent imperviousness and immutability to, for example, HFA 2000 and a reorientation of services to PHC, with consequences for roles for staff and their education and training. Professional training across all groups appears to have followed the route of specialisation to a point of overkill (WHO, 1985c).

Despite such negative remarks, in terms of the two arenas of production and management, the NHS is at least at face value seeking to achieve the objectives depicted in the evaluative checklist. But as for the planning dimension, a different conceptual viewpoint is required. The notions of 'teams', 'their composition', and 'levels of health' and the interlinking of such concepts seem alien in the NHS. They do not figure in discussions in the professional literature, Health Authority manpower plans, or the postal questionnaire responses. In contrast, the planning dimension is phrased in terms of 'getting the right people with the right qualificatons at the right time'. A 'numbers' orientation abounds, which becomes translated into an occupationally based approach. Forecasts of doctors and nurses are undertaken, and shortages of physiotherapists noted. Accordingly, issues such as role questionning and definition, interprofessional collaboration and working in multidisciplinary teams towards the achievement of specified health objectives are not the coinage of current manpower practice. There are of course exceptions: for example, Project 2000 in relation to the role of the nurse; teamworking in schemes for the care of the elderly, mental illness and mental handicap; and team working in primary health care. Interestingly perhaps, such instances involve a context where the physician is perceived as one amongst many with specialist expertise, and not as the dominant player.

Within the NHS, the objective of the planning dimension is alternatively defined as being 'to specify the number of staff required', a narrower and more restricted statement with potential for accepting the status quo as the pattern for the future. Role questioning, close examination of manpower patterns and skill mixes in relation to health needs and demands, or attempts to influence the production dimension are unlikely to occur. Outside of nursing, few such examples are apparent. In contrast, medical dominance and attempts by other groups to establish an acknowledged professional status can be observed; and within forecasts of staffing numbers, current role definitions are seemingly assumed. But at least manpower is seen as a major element in planning - having recently advanced from little more than an afterthought.

Even more fundamentally, the basic problem may be that the NHS has a lack of commitment to planning in general and the manpower dimension in particular. Strategic planning, begun in 1976, had not really got off the ground before control, costs containment and efficiency savings became the modus operandi. Further, it has not been based on clear objectives linked to the community's health; indeed, explicit objectives for the NHS are hard to find (Royal Commission on the NHS Report, 1979). Plans have thus played a more symbolic role than actually indicating a true direction for service development.

Finally, in terms of the integration of the three dimensions of the health manpower process, the main thrust has been on costs. Attempts to influence the production sector, to achieve a workforce possessing appropriate education and training, have been little pursued. But given the lack of clarity over (health) objectives, it is not surprising that the management dimension of the health manpower process has been dominant.

INNOVATION IN MANPOWER PRACTICE

A negative picture has been presented in applying the evaluative checklist elaborated in Table 12.1 to NHS manpower practices, at least as the latter emerged in the survey and the study of the professional literature. However, there are many instances of patterns of manpower organisation and working relationships that belie this evaluative description. It is to a consideration of factors facilitating and preventing these 'innovatory' manpower practices, and also to the potential for their diffusion that discusson now turns.

The case study of the manpower issues surrounding the transition of care for the mentally handicapped from hospital to community, alone of the three, provides an illustration of the opportunities for the planning of the service and its manpower to affect the production and management dimensions of the health manpower process. It is too early to say whether such a possibility for integrating the manpower dimensions will be realised; for implementation of the service plan has not yet occurred. Further changes on the production side will be more slow in emerging; notwithstanding, the ENB (1982) has outlined courses for nurses of relevance to this transition. But the major immediate impact is likely to occur within the management dimension, in order to make the service operate at all.

What factors stimulated this service change, and the consequent reassessment of manpower skills, roles and requirements? Firstly, there was the encouragement of the central Health Departments in numerous policy documents dating back at least to the 1971 White Paper (DHSS, 1971). It too fits well with broader health care notions as, for example, HFA 2000 and a reorientation of services towards PHC. Secondly, public opinion, while often showing itself as unhappy with the precise location of community based hostels, has also become opposed to the existence of large, isolated mental institutions. Thirdly, given central support, resource allocations for the changeover in service provision have been supportive, at least until local authority social services experienced difficulties over cash limits in recent years.

The major health services problem has been that relating to manpower - what will happen to the registered mental handicap nurses? Will they become hostel workers, or are they, as it were, themselves

237

victims of the long stay institution and unable to adapt to the different community situation? A major manpower issue is thus presented. In terms of the evaluative discussion above, role questionning and exploration had to occur, consideration to be given to the possible transfer (through continuing education) of 'old' into 'new' skills, the very difficulty posed by professionalism to be examined, and multidisciplinary, and inter-sectoral (health and health-related) teams to be developed to provide the services. It must also be noted that physicians are not the pre-eminent health care practitioners with regard to the mentally handicapped; this has probably facilitated the movement towards inter-professional collaboration, and a rejection of over-specialisation. Indeed, both their, and the nurses' roles and professionalism came under scrutiny because of the new caring context.

The changes in mental handicap services are in their early stages and many of the manpower issues remain to be addressed, let alone resolved. The case study itself represented only the initial approach of one Health Authority. Its experiences, while differing somewhat in their detail, can be replicated across the NHS. The transfer of the mental handicapped to the community has been widely promoted for its general merit. What continues to be of critical interest is the extent to which role questionning, inter-professional collaboration and the like leads onto a deployment of manpower of direct benefit to patient health, and also the degree of influence which new or modified manpower utilisation patterns will exert on the education and training of future staff.

Both the health centre and the study of nurses in PHC exemplify the management dimension of the health manpower process. While health centres have been officially commended, in terms of the possibility of purpose-built accommodation with rent and rates paid, and also for the opportunities to employ ancillary staff (and recover 70% of their cost), and for the attachment of Health Authority nursing staff, there is little evidence of explicit attempts to 'plan' manpower or facilities. Further, the production sector appears to have been slowly attracted by the notion of PHC; it is only in the last ten years that GPs have emerged out of the shadow of their consultant colleagues; a similar story applies in nursing.

In terms of facilitating PHC, and associated multidisciplinary, and again inter-sectoral, teams

it has has been left in the hands of individual GPs
for the most part. The recent Green Paper (DHSS,
1986b) itself, while advocating a 'good practice
allowance', does not suggest that 'poor practices'
might be equally directly penalised. The Green
Paper also declines to draw any connections between
its own schemes for fees and allowances to widen
a GP's activities, and the RCGP (1985) initiatives
towards 'good quality' payments which it also warmly
endorses.

For the nurse in the PHC context, and in
particular, the nurse practitioner role, any such
development at the present time lies in the hands
of interested GPs. There is an obvious incentive
to employ a practice nurse, especially as the extra
fees generated will almost certainly more than cover
the cost to the GP, and because the physician has
a control over such nurses which is less certain
with attached staff. A nurse practitioner may be
employed on the same financial arrangements as a
practice nurse - but with a different role agreed.
In terms of the production dimension, the post-
basic qualifications for practice nurses are a
matter for debate, and even more mystery surrounds
the training required for a role such as that
performed by Stilwell (1982a). The RCN (1984) has
proposed some training, as too have GPs (Mourin,
1980), but otherwise it is again left to interested
individuals to arrange. Before 1986, this manpower
innovation was treated askance by both the majority
of doctors and nurses. Whether the positive support
for the nurse practitioner role in the Cumberlege
Report (DHSS, 1986a) will lead to the development
of special training 'pre' or 'post' qualification
remains to be seen; the UKCC Project 2000 Report
(1986) sketches out its preferred line of growth.
In terms of the evaluation of manpower practice a
major question mark is raised over the issue of
professionalism and autonomy, and thus
specialisation. The seeds of an expansion from the
role of a 'traditional' nurse to a more enlarged,
and different role are nevertheless being actively
sown at the present time. What is uncertain is how
far any moves towards a holistic approach to health
care, with an emphasis on prevention, counselling
and treatment, will instead nurture new specialisms
within nursing.

These case studies illustrate some of the ways
in which the establishment and diffusion of manpower
practices associated with PHC are (not) carried
forward. Most of the innovative work owes little

to the monitoring and review procedures inaugurated by the DHSS. There is a certain flexibility in NHS working relations which allows scope for committed individuals (particularly physicians) to introduce changes. The wider diffusion of 'good practice' is only possible if support is forthcoming from Health Authorities and professional associations. The survey results highlighted the central pressure on Authorities to evaluate plans in terms of affordability, performance indicators, and guarantees about staff supply. The general climate in the NHS has been of increasing economic uncertainty and this has encouraged a conservatism in health manpower practices rather than acting as a catalyst for significant changes.

The move towards PHC demonstrates a constellation of the factors associated with an 'implementation failure' (Gray and Hunter, 1983). There is widespread ambiguity in the commitment to PHC, which threatens to become all things to all people. While it has been sometimes promoted as a less costly alternative, the information on which this is based is far from convincing. Further, it ignores the ambitions of those who anticipate a marked expansion in health promotion, prevention and community services far beyond their present levels. It is doubtful therefore how far political support will stand firm in the face of increased demands for resources.

Given the breadth of interpretation of what PHC comprises, it is likely to become something of a battleground between competing professionals. The current emphasis in the NHS on 'headcounts' suggests that the evaluation techniques have done little to reorient management or professionals to the effectiveness of different manpower mixes or practices. By the same token, manpower production remains resolutely outside management control, and the professionals have sought to extend formal education and training rather than give more weight to 'on-the-job' training.

The picture of the health manpower process outlined here does not accord well with the rationalist model of decision making. The particular encouragement of PHC practices requires support or at least non-opposition across the health services from the major interest groups. The processes of monitoring and review have not given the sure capability for the centre to over-ride local or professional opposition - for example, the saga of consultant numbers. At the same time, the medical profession cannot afford to disregard opposition from Health Authorities and the DHSS. There are in the NHS many opportunities and interests willing and able to veto policies which might take the NHS in new directions (Klein, 1983).

The setting seems conducive to 'illuminative' evaluation rather than that proposed in the rational model (Carr-Hill, 1985, p. 372). This implies something of a return to an 'incrementalist' approach. It bears witness to the complexities of decision making in the NHS (Illsley, 1980; Klein and O'Higgins, 1985). The difficulty for the health manpower process is that while forward planning - such as the extension of PHC in HFA 2000 - is a necessary exercise, it cannot rest on the rationalist procedures currently emphasised in official accounts. Th alternative course is to plan for changing circumstances, but also to provide sufficient flexibility in both procedures and objectives for health manpower, that will offer some opportunity for better adaptation to an uncertain future.

APPENDIX

POSTAL QUESTIONNAIRE

I would be grateful if you would spare some
time to answer the following questions which explore
the way manpower requirements are formulated, the
match between supply and demand, and strategies
which you may have tried and adopted to influence
the supply of labour.

The questions are designed to be answered by
ticking the appropriate category. In addition, I
would like you to amplify your responses where
appropriate in as much detail as possible.

Thank you for your help.

A STAFFING REQUIREMENTS

1 There are many different methods for estimating
   the requirements for staff. Which of the
   following do you use? If you are using a
   combination of methods please indicate one.

   (For allied health professionals and personnel)

           Professional judgement   ...
           Norms (please indicate which
             norms you use)   ...
           Workload based method - please
             elaborate   ...
           Other - please specify   ...

   (For nurses)

           Professional judgement   ...
           Norms (please indicate which
             norms you use)   ...
           Telford formula   ...
           Cheltenham method   ...
           Goddard method   ...

242

        Leicester method   ...
        Oxfordshire method   ...
        Rhys Hearn Care Package   ...
        Aberdeen formula   ...
        Auld method   ...
        Other - please specify   ...

2 Please can you tell me why you have adopted this
   particular method(s).

3 What advantages and disadvantages have you found
   in this approach? Please give as much detail as
   you can.

4 Do ·you intend to change your method of estimating
   staffing requirements in the near future?

   YES   NO

   If so, which method will you be changing to, and
   why?

5 In your experience, is the estimation of the
   demand for your staff undertaken on a staff group
   by staff group basis (ie, for nurses, doctors,
   and physiotherapists, etc, independently of each
   other)?

        Totally   ...
        To a large extent   ...
        To some extent   ...
        Not at all   ...
        Don't know   ...

   Why do you say this?

6 An alternative approach to this is that of
   planning staffing requirements across groups,
   and looking at the joint contribution staff
   groups (as a multiprofessional team) make to
   patient care. To what extent has such an
   approach been operating in your area of
   activity?

   1 Useful approach, and has been
         adopted   ...
   2 Useful approach, and starting
         to do things in this way   ...

3 Useful approach, and would hope
  to pursue it in the near
  future   ...
4 Unacceptable option, tried in
  the past but did not work   ...
5 Unacceptable option - please
  explain   ...
6 Don't know   ...

What is the reason for your view?

B   LABOUR SUPPLY

7 Have you ever experienced any problems in recruiting staff?

    Never   ...
    Occasionally   ...
    Frequently   ...
    Most of the time   ...
    Don't know   ...

If so, which particular grades of staff did you
find it difficult to recruit, and why do you
think that was?

8 Which of the following strategies have you
  employed in attempting to overcome labour
  supply difficulties? Please tick those
  which you have tried.

                              YES NO

    Advertising campaign (to
      "sell" the district, showing
      its attractiveness)   ... ...
    Mounting a back to "nursing"
      campaign   ... ...
    Register of ex-employees
      (eg, nurse bank)   ... ...
    Undertake a labour market
      survey, to explore the
      possible sources of recruits ... ...
    Attracting more people to
      take up training places   ... ...
    Opening and/or expanding
      training school   ... ...
    Upgrading posts   ... ...
    Offering a higher salary/in-
      cremental starting point   ... ...

Increasing openings for
  part-time employment   ... ...
Providing creche facilities   ... ...
Enlarging the role of a member
  of staff to embrace the
  shortage skill   ... ...
Changing the staffing mix   ... ...
Retraining existing staff to
  take on additional skills
  in the shortage area   ... ...
Other - please specify   ... ...
None of these, as the supply
  of labour was never a problem ... ...

Does this combination of strategies work successfully to solve the supply problem?

YES   NO

Why do you say this?

Finally, which of these do you think was most successful, and why?

C MANPOWER PLANNING ROLE

9 Do you feel that the introduction of manpower targets since 1983 has overridden manpower planning, in the since of formulating staffing requirements and ensuring supply is achieved?

Completely   ...
Partly   ...
Not at all   ...
Not sure   ...

Why do you think so, and how has it effected this?

10 Is there a vacancy review procedure operating in the District?

YES   NO

If so, what criteria must be satisfied in order to make a case of need, to fill a vacant post?

11 Has the RHA provided you with any advice, guidelines or support in developing the manpower
contribution to the current (1984-1994) Strategic
Plan?

YES   NO

If so, how has it helped you?

12 What role do you personally play in manpower
planning?

   i   Advisory and consultative   ...
   ii   Formulating staffing require-
        ments only   ...
   iii Formulating staffing require-
        ments and ensuring supply are
        achieved   ...
   iv   Ensuring supply only is achieved   ...

If (i) or (ii), who pursued the issues of ensuring the supply of manpower?

13 Finally, the World Health Organisation describes
the objective of health manpower planning as
being 'to specify the number of teams and the
composition needed to improve the level of health
up to a proposed level'. Does this describe what
you currently do?

YES   NO

Please can you tell me why you say this?

Thank you for completing this questionnaire.

Please return the completed questionnaire in the
pre-addressed envelope.

BIBLIOGRAPHY

Alford, R. (1975) Health Care Politics, University of
    Chicago Press, Chicago
Allen, D.E. (1979) Hospital Planning: the Development
    of the 1962 Hospital Plan, Pitman Medical,
    Tunbridge Wells
Allen, M. (1986) 'Medical unemployment - fact or
    fiction?', Health Services Manpower Review, Vol.
    11, No. 4, pp. 6-7
All Wales Nurse Manpower Planning Committee (1985)
    First Report, Welsh Office, Cardiff
Appleyard, W.J. (1982) 'Medical manpower: mirage or
    miracle?', British Medical Journal, Vol. 284, 1
    May, pp. 1351-1355
Armitage, D. (1983) 'Joint working in primary health
    care', Nursing Times, Occasional Papers 79, pp.
    75-78
Armstrong, D. (1976) 'The decline of medical hegemony:
    a review of government reports during the NHS',
    Social Science and Medicine, Vol. 10, pp. 157-63
Balint, M. (1968, 1980 second ed.) The Doctor,
    His Patient and the Illness, Oxford University
    Press, London
Bankowski, Z. and Bryant, J.H. (eds.) (1983) Health
    For All - A Challenge to Research in Health
    Manpower Development, Council for International
    Organisations of Medical Sciences, Geneva
Bayley, M. (1973) Mental Handicap and Community Care,
    Routledge and Kegan Paul, London
Bendall, E. (1985) 'Strategy for Change', Senior
    Nurse, Vol. 3, No. 2, July, p. 53
Bevan, R.G. and Spencer, A.H. (1984) 'Models of
    resources policy of regional authorities', in M.
    Clarke (ed.) Planning Analysis in Health Care
    Systems, Pion, London, pp. 90-118
Birch, S. and Maynard, A. (1985) 'Dental manpower',
    Social Policy and Administration, Vol. 19, No. 3,
    pp. 199-217

Bibliography

Bloore, J. (1984) 'Manpower planning two: a system from Gloucestershire', Nursing Times, 22 August, pp. 55-7

Bolt, D.E. (1983) 'Medical manpower in the year 2000', British Medical Association, London

Bond, J. et al (1985) A Study of Interprofessional Collaboration in Primary Health Care Organisations, Vol. II, Report No. 27, Health Care Research Unit, University of Newcastle Upon Tyne

Bosanquet, N. and Gerard, N. (1985) Nurse Manpower: Recent Trends and Policy Options, Discussion Paper 9, Centre for Health Economics, University of York

Bowling, A. (1981) Delegation in General Practice: A Study of Doctors and Nurses, Tavistock, London

Bowling, A. (1985a) 'Which tasks can a community nurse take over?', Nursing Times, 23 October, pp. 46-47

Bowling, A. (1985b) 'Doctors and nurses: delegation and substitution' in A. Harrison and J. Gretton (eds.) Health Care UK 1985, Chartered Institute of Public Finance and Accountancy, London, pp. 59-67

Boylan, A. (1982) 'Nursing at the crossroads: the role of the nurse in the future', Nursing Mirror, Vol. 78, 15 September, pp. 161-163

Brearley, S. (1984) 'The medical manpower crisis - who can solve it?' Health Services Manpower Review, Vol. 10, No. 2, pp. 8-10

Briggs Report (1972) Report of the Committee on Nursing, Cmnd. 5115, HMSO, London

Briggs, P.J., Fletcher, P., Popplewell, R. and Riley, B.B. (1980) 'Relationship between patient data and pharmacy workload and staffing', Pharmaceutical Journal, Vol. 224, pp. 282-4

British Dental Association (1982) Dental Manpower Requirements to 2020, BDA, London

British Dental Journal (1983) 'Fewer but taught longer', Editorial, Vol. 154, 19 February, p. 91

British Medical Association (1983) General practice - a British Success, General Medical Services Committee, British Medical Association, London

British Medical Journal (1985) 'Immigration rules to apply to doctors', Vol. 290, 6 April, p. 1087

Brooker, C. and Beard, P. (1984) 'The nursing alternative', Senior Nurse, Vol. 1, No. 36, 5 December, pp. 14-17

Bibliography

Brown, A.M. et al (1986) 'The future of general practitioners in Newcastle Upon Tyne', Lancet, 15 February, pp. 370-71

Buchan, J. (1985) 'What happened to the chiefs?', Nursing Times, 6 November, pp. 24-6

Busuttil, J. (1985) 'Community occupational therapy and the general practitioner', Occupational Therapy, March, pp. 80-2

Butler, J.R. and Vaile, S.B. (1984) Health and Social Services, Routledge and Kegan Paul, London

Campion, P.D. (1985) 'Setting standards in general practice', British Medical Journal, Vol. 291, 25 August, p. 499

Carr, T.E.A. (1979) 'Whither general practice?', Health Trends, Vol. 11, No. 4, pp. 83-8

Carr-Hill, R.A., (1985) 'The evaluation of health care', Social Science and Medicine, Vol. 2, No. 4, pp. 367-375

Carruthers, I.J. (1984) 'Medical manpower planning - a view from a district', Hospital and Health Services Review, Vol. 80, No. 6, pp. 286-8

Cartwright, A. and Anderson, R. (1981) General Practice Revisited, Tavistock, London

Central Statistical Office (1984) Regional Trends 1984, HMSO, London

Chaplin, N. (ed.) (1982) Health Care in the United Kingdom: Its Organisation and Management, Kluwer Medical, London

Chartered Society of Physiotherapy (1984) District Physiotherapy Management: Why It Must Stay, CSP Briefing Paper No. 3, CSP, London

Chartered Society of Physiotherapy (1986) 'Physiotherapy, chiropody, occupational therapy and allied fields of study in public sector education', Physiotherapy, Vol. 72, No. 2, pp. 79-80

Cohen, P. (1984) 'Nurse practitioner in East London',Nursing Times, 11 January, pp. 22-24

College of Occupational Therapists (1980) Recommended Minimum Standards for Occupational Therapy Staff: Patient Ratios, London

Council for Professions Supplementary to Medicine (1977) PSM Education and Training: the Next Decade, CPSM, London

Council for Professions Supplementary to Medicine (1980a) Annual Report, 1979/80, London

Council for Professions Supplementary to Medicine (1980b) PSM Registration and Self-Regulation: Future Requirements and Opportunities, CPSM, London

Bibliography

Council for Professions Supplementary to Medicine
(1981) Annual Report 1980/81, London
Council for Professions Supplementary to Medicine
(1983a) New Working Party on Chiropodial Surgical
Practice, Press Statement, 23 March
Council for Professions Supplementary to Medicine
(1983b) Independent Inquiry, Press Release, 28
October
Council for Professions Supplementary to Medicine
(1984) Proposed Merger of Physiotherapists and
Remedial Gymnasts' Boards, Press Statement, 18
April
Council for Professions Supplementary to Medicine
(1985) Annual Report 1984/5, CPSM, London
Coyne, A-M., (1985) 'Manpower planning in practice',
Health and Social Service Journal, 3 October, p.
1230
Cree, J. (1981) 'Manpower information system', in A.F.
Long and G. Mercer (eds) Manpower Planning in the
National Health Service, London, ch. 4
Crossman, R.H.S. (1972) A Politician's View of Health
Service Planning, University of Glasgow Press,
Glasgow
Dawe, A. (1984) 'You and your profession', Nursing
Mirror, Vol. 158, 3 May, pp. 28-30
Dawson Report (1920) Consultative Council on Medical
and Allied Services, Report on the Future
Provision of Medical and Allied Services, HMSO,
London
Day, P. and Klein, R. (1985) 'Central accountability
and local decision-making: towards a new NHS',
British Medical Journal, Vol. 290, pp. 1676-1678
Department of Health and Social Security (1956) Report
of the Committee on Recruitment to the Dental
Profession (McNair Report), Cmnd. 9861, HMSO,
London
Department of Health and Social Security (1971) Better
Services for the Mentally Handicapped, Cmnd.
4683, HMSO, London
Department of Health and Social Security (1972)
Management Arrangements for the Reorganised
National Health Service, DHSS, London
Department of Health and Social Security (1973)
Report of a Working Party on the Remedial
Professions, (McMillan Report), DHSS, London
Department of Health and Social Security (1974)
Democracy in the National Health Service, HMSO,
London

Bibliography

Department of Health and Social Security (1975) Report
    of the Committee of Inquiry Into the Pay and
    Related Conditions of Service of the Professions
    Supplementary to Medicine and Speech Therapists,
    (Halsbury Report), HMSO, London
Department of Health and Social Security (1976a) The
    NHS Planning System, DHSS, London
Department of Health and Social Security (1976b)
    Priorities for Health and Personal Social
    Services in England: A Consultative Document,
    HMSO, London
Department of Health and Social Security (1976c)
    Sharing Resources for Health in England, the
    Report of the Resource Allocation Working Party,
    HMSO, London
Department of Health and Social Security (1977) Health
    Services Development: Relationship Between the
    Medical and the Remedial Professions, HC(77)33,
    DHSS, London
Department of Health and Social Security (1978)
    Medical Manpower - The Next Twenty Years, HMSO,
    London
Department of Health and Social Security (1979a)
    Patients First, HMSO, London
Department of Health and Social Security (1979b)
    Report of the Committee of Enquiry into Mental
    Handicap Nursing and Care, Cmnd. 7468, HMSO,
    London
Department of Health and Social Security (1980a)
    Report of the Medical Manpower Steering Group,
    DHSS, London
Department of Health and Social Security (1980b)
    Supply of and Demand for Occupational Therapists
    Working in the NHS in Great Britain, Dear
    Administrator Letter, DA(80)10
Department of Health and Social Security (1980c)
    Mental Handicap: Progress, Problems and
    Priorities, DHSS, London
Department of Health and Social Security (1981a) Care
    in Action: A Handbook of Policies and Priorities
    for Health and Personal Social Services in
    England, HMSO, London
Department of Health and Social Security (1981b) Care
    in the Community, a Consultative Document on
    Moving Resources for Care in England, DHSS,
    London
Department of Health and Social Security (1981c)
    Staffing in the Remedial Professions: A Study,
    Central Management Services, London

Department of Health and Social Security (1982), Government Response to the Fourth Report From the Social Servies Committee 1980-81 Session, Cmnd. 8479, HMSO, London

Department of Health and Social Security (1982a) Nurse Manpower: Maintaining the Balance, DHSS, London

Department of Health and Social Security (1983a) Health Service Management Performance Indicators, HN(83)25, DHSS, London

Department of Health and Social Security (1983b) Dental Manpower, Report of the Department Study Group on Dental Manpower, HMSO, London

Department of Health and Social Security (1983c) NHS Management Inquiry (Letter to Secretary of State) (Griffiths Report), DHSS, London

Department of Health and Social Security (1983d) Nurse Manpower Planning: Approaches and Techniques, HMSO, London

Department of Health and Social Security (1984a) Nurse Manpower Project for NHS Management Inquiry, HMSO, London

Department of Health and Social Security (1984b) Report of the Joint Working Group on Collaboration between Family Practitioners and District Health Authorities, DHSS, London

Department of Health and Social Security (1984c) The Health Service in England, Annual Report 1984, DHSS, London

Department of Health and Social Security (1985a) Report of the Advisory Committee for Medical Manpower Planning, DHSS, London

Department of Health and Social Security (1985b) Community Care: With Special Reference to Adult Mentally Ill and Mentally Handicapped People, Cmnd. 9674, HMSO, London

Department of Health and Social Security (1986a) Neighbourhood Nursing - A Focus for Care, (Cumberlege Report), HMSO

Department of Health and Social Security (1986b) Primary Health Care: An Agenda for Discussion, Cmnd. 9771, DHSS, London

Dickson, N. (1985) 'Project 2000. Pointing a way forward', Nursing Times, 4 December, pp. 26-28

Dingwall, R. and McIntosh, J. (eds.) (1978) Readings in the Sociology of Nursing, Churchill Livingstone, Edinburgh

Donald, B.L. (1981) 'Health care professionalism: reinforcement required?', Social Policy and Administration, Vol. 15, No. 3, pp. 242-257

Bibliography

Dowson, S. and Maynard, A. (1985) 'General practice', in A. Morrison and J. Gretton (eds.) Health Care UK 1985, Chartered Institute of Public Finance and Accountancy, London, pp. 15-26

Doyal, L. and Epstein, S.E. (1983) Cancer in Britain: The Politics of Prevention, Pluto Press, London

Draper, J. (1981) 'From handmaiden to health specialist', Nursing Mirror, 24 June, pp. 22-24

Dunnell, K. and Dobbs, J. (1982) Nurses Working in the Community, OPCS, HMSO, London

English National Board (1982) Syllabus of Training: Professional Register Part 5, (Registered Nurse for the Mentally Handicapped), ENB, London

English National Board (1985a) Professional Education/Training Courses, ENB, London

English National Board (1985b) Education and Training of Nurses Caring for People with Mental Handicap, Circular 1985/55/ERDB, ENB, London

Etzioni, A. (1967) 'Mixed scanning: a "third" approach to decision making', Public Administration Review, Vol. 27, pp. 385-392

Farrow, G. (1982) 'A nurse bank with built-in training', Nursing Times, 19 May, pp. 855-857

Feinmann, J. (1985) 'An experiment paying dividends',Health and Social Service Journal, 3 October, pp. 1228-1229

Feinmann, J. (1986) 'Power struggle for FPCs', Health and Social Service Journal, 6 March, pp. 306-307

Ferlie, E., Pahl, J. and Quine, L. (1984) 'Professional collaboration in services for mentally handicapped people', Journal of Social Policy, Vol. 13, pp. 185-202

Finch, J and Groves, D. (1980) 'Community care and the family: a case for equal opportunities?', Journal of Social Policy, Vol. 9, No. 4, pp. 496-509

Fry, J. (1983) Present State and Future Needs in General Practice, Royal College of General Practitioners, MTP Press, Lancaster

Fry, J. and Hasler, J.C. (1986) Primary Health Care 2000, Churchill Livingstone, Edinburgh

Fullard, E., Fowles, G. and Muir Gray (1984) 'Facilitating prevention in primary care', British Medical Journal, Vol. 289, 8 December, pp. 1585-1587

Fulop, T. (1976) 'New approach to an old problem: the case of health services', WHO Chronicle, 30, pp. 433-441

Bibliography

Fulop, T. (1980) 'The health services and manpower development concept - health manpower: for what?', in H. Noack (ed.) Medical Education and Primary Health Care, Croom Helm, London, ch. 1

Fulop, T. (1982) 'The future of WHO's health manpower development programme, WHO Chronicle, Vol. 36, No. 1, pp. 3-6

Gaze, H. (1986) 'Out in the cold', Nursing Times, 27 February, pp. 18-19

Gilmore, M., Bruce, N. and Hunt, M. (1974) The Work of the Nursing Team in General Practice, Council for the Education and Training of Health Visitors, London

Gladstone, D. (1982) 'Community, co-ordination and collaboration: some themes in policy for the mentally handicapped', in C. Jones and J. Stevenson (eds.) The Year Book of Social Policy in Britain 1980-81, Routledge and Kegan Paul, London, ch. 10

Glennerster, H. (1981) 'From containment to conflict? Social planning in the seventies', Journal of Social Policy, Vol. 10, No. 1, pp. 31-51

Glennerster, H. (1983) Planning for Priority Groups, Martin Roberston, Oxford

Goodenough Report (1944) Report of the Inter Departmental Committee on Medical Schools, Ministry of Health, London

Gray, A.M. and Hunter, D.J. (1983) 'Priorities and resource allocation in the Scottish health services', Policy and Politics, Vol. 11, No. 4, pp. 417-437

Green, A. and Rathwell, T. (1985) 'Planning family practitioner services', Hospital and Health Services Review, Vol. 81, No. 1, pp. 14-16

Guillebaud Report (1956) Report of the Committee of Enquiry into the Cost of the National Health Service, Cmnd. 9663, HMSO, London

Hall, T.L. and Mejia, A. (eds.) (1978) Health Manpower Planning: Principles, Methods and Issues, WHO, Geneva

Halsbury Report (1975) Committee of Enquiry into the Pay and Related Conditions of Service of the Professions Supplementary to Medicine and Speech Therapists Report, HMSO, London

Ham, C. (1981) Policy Making in the NHS, Macmillan, London

Harding Report (1981) The Primary Health Care Team. Report of a Joint Working Group of the Standing Advisory Committee and the Standing Nursing and Midwifery Advisory Committee, DHSS, London

Bibliography

Harrison, S. (1981) 'The politics of health manpower', in A.F. Long and G. Mercer (eds.) Manpower Planning in the National Health Service, Gower, Farnborough, ch. 5

Harrison, S. (1985) 'Perspectives on implementation', in A.F. Long and S. Harrison (eds.) Health Services Performance: Effectiveness and Efficiency, Croom Helm, London, ch. 5

Harrison, S. (1987) 'Health care in Great Britain', in R.B. Saltman (ed.) International Handbook of Health Care Systems, Greenwood Press, Westport, USA

Harrison, S. and Henly, J. (1982) 'Remedial professions: lines of accountability', Health and Social Service Journal, 22 April, pp. 505-508

Harrison, S. and Brooks, F. (1985) Professional Manpower in the Yorkshire Region, Nuffield Centre, University of Leeds

Hart, J.T. (1985a) 'Practice nurses: an underused resource', British Medical Journal, Vol. 290, 20 April, pp. 1162-1163

Hart, J.T. (1985b) 'When practice is not perfect', Nursing Times, 25 September, pp. 28-29

Haywood, S. (1983) 'The politics of management in health care: A British perspective', Journal of Health Politics, Policy and Law, Vol. 8, No. 3, pp. 424-443

Haywood, S. and Alaszewski, A. (1979) Crisis in the Health Service, Croom Helm, London

Haywood, S. and Hunter, D.J. (1982) 'Consultative processes in health policy in the United Kingdom: a view from the centre', Public Administration, Vol. 69, Summer, pp. 143-162

Health Circular HC(77)33, Health Services Development: Relationship between the Medical and Remedial Professions, DHSS, September 1980

Health Circular HC(79)8, Health Services Development: Primary Health Care, Health Centres and Other Premises, DHSS, April 1979

Health Circular HC(82)4, Health Services Management: Hospital Medical Staff, Career Structure and Training, DHSS, February 1982

Health Circular HC(82)6, The NHS Planning System, DHSS, March, 1982

Health Circular HC(82)14, Health Services Development: Resource Assumptions and Planning Guidelines in 1982-83 to 1984-85, DHSS, July 1982

Bibliography

Health Circular HC(83)4, Health Services Development:
     Resources Allocation for 1983/84, DHSS, January
     1983
Health Circular HC(83)16, Cash Limits and Manpower
     Targets for 1983-84, DHSS, August 1983
Health Circular HC(83)25, Health Service Management
     Performance Indicators, DHSS, September 1983
Health Circular HC(84)2, Resource Distribution for
     1984-85, Service Priorities, Manpower and
     Planning, DHSS, January 1984
Health Circular HC(84)10, Health Services Development:
     Reports of the Steering Group on Health Services
     Information: Implementation Programme, DHSS, Apri
     1984
Health Circular HC(84)13, Implementation of the NHS
     Management Inquiry Report, DHSS, June 1984
Hicks, D. (1976) Primary Health Care, HMSO, London
Hill, D.M. (1979) 'Evaluation in policy making:
     the case of structure planning', Public
     Administration Bulletin, No. 30, August, pp. 23-
     46
Hirschorn, L. (1980) 'Scenario writing: a development
     approach', Journal of the American Planning
     Association, Vol. 45, No. 2, pp. 172-182
Hodder Report (1943) Report of the Nursing
     Reconstruction Committee, RCN, London
Hofoss, D. (1980) 'Health professions: the origin of
     species', Social Science and Medicine, Vol. 22,
     No. 2, pp. 201-207
Honigsbaum, F. (1979) The Division in British
     Medicine, Kogan Page, London
Horder, J.P. (1985) 'The balance between primary and
     secondary care - a personal view', Health Trends,
     Vol. 17, pp. 64-68
House of Commons Social Services Committee (1981)
     Fourth Report of the Social Services Committee
     1980-8. Medical Education with Special Reference
     to the Number of Doctors and the Career Structure
     in Hospitals, (the Short Report), HMSO, London
House of Commons (1985a) Fifth Report from the Social
     Services Committee. Medical Education Report:
     Follow-Up, HMSO, London
House of Commons (1985b) Second Report from the
     Social Services Committee, 1984-85, Community
     Care, HMSO, London
Hunter, D.J. (1983) 'Centre-periphery relations in the
     National Health Service: facilitators or
     inhibitors of innovation?', in K. Young (ed.)
     National Interests and Local Government,
     Heinemann, London, ch. 7

Bibliography

Hutt, R. (1984) 'Training and jobs', Nursing Times, 14
     March, pp. 47-52
Illsley, R. (1980) Professional or Public Health?
     Nuffield Provincial Hospitals Trust, London
Illsley, V. and Goldstone, L. (1985) 'Methods of
     planning', Senior Nurse, Vol. 3, No. 6, pp. 14-
     18
Jack, A.B. and Alpine, R.L.W. (1980) 'Optical
     services in the UK: a study of a professional
     labour market', Omega, Vol. 8, No. 6, pp. 681-9
Jameson Report (1956) An Inquiry into Health
     Visiting, HMSO, London
Jarman, B. (1983) 'Identification of
     underprivileged areas', British Medical Journal,
     Vol. 288, 11 February, pp. 1705-1709
Jay Report (1979) Report of the Committee of
     Inquiry into Mental Handicap Nursing and Care,
     Cmnd. 7468, Vols I and II, HMSO, London
Jefferys, M. and Sachs, H. (1983) Rethinking
     General Practice: Dilemmas in Primary Medical
     Care, Tavistock, London
Kaprio, L.A. (1979) Primary Health Care in
     Europe, WHO, Copenhagen
Klein, R. (1982) 'Performance, evaluation and the
     NHS: a case study in conceptual perplexity and
     organisational complexity', Public
     Administration, Vol. 60, No. 4, pp. 385-407
Klein, R. (1983) The Politics of the National Health
     Service, Longman, Harlow
Klein, R. and O'Higgins, M. (eds.) (1985) The Future
     of Welfare, Basil Blackwell, Oxford
Kohn, R. (1983) 'The health centre concept in primary
     health care', Public Health in Europe, 22, WHO,
     Copenhagen
Korner, E. (1984) Third Report to the Secretary of
     State: A Report on the Collection and Use of
     Information about Manpower in the NHS, HMSO,
     London
Kratz, C. (1985) 'Nurse of all trades?', Nursing
     Times, 4 December, pp. 32-33
Larkin, G.V. (1983) Occupational Monopoly and Modern
     Medicine, Tavistock, London
Lewis, J. and Brookes, B. (1983) 'The Peckham health
     Centre, "pep", and the concept of general
     practice during the 1930s and 1940s', Medical
     History, Vol. 27, pp. 151-161
Lindblom, C.E. (1959) 'The science of muddling
     through', Public Administration, Vol. 19, pp. 79-
     88

Lindblom, C.E. (1979) 'Still muddling, not yet through', Public Administration, Vol. 39, pp. 517-526

Lind, G. and Wiseman, C. (1978) 'Setting Health priorities: a review of concepts and approaches', Journal of Social Policy, Vol. 7, No. 4, pp. 411-440

Linstead, D. (1984) 'The realities of human resourcing: a case study of the utility of rational planning models in health care', Health Services Manpower Review, Vol. 10, No. 3, pp. 9-11

London Health Planning Consortium (1981) Primary Health Care in Inner London, (Acheson Report), London

Long, A.F. and Mercer, G. (1978) 'Nurses down the drain?', Nursing Mirror, Vol. 147, 23 November, pp. 16-18

Long, A.F. and Mercer, G. (eds.) (1981) Manpower Planning in the National Health Service, Gower, Farnborough

Long, A.F. and Harrison, S. (eds.) (1985) Health Services Performance: Effectiveness and Efficiency, Croom Helm, London

Long, A.F., Harrison, S., Greenwood, N., Henderson, J., and Hodgson, P. (1983) Characteristics of NHS Administrators: Report on the 1979 Survey, DHSS, London

McCarthy, M. (1983) 'Are efficiency measures effective?', Health and Social Service Journal, 15 December, pp. 1500-1501

McCormick, J. (1979) The Doctor: Father Figure or Plumber?, Croom Helm, London

Majone, G. and Wildavsky, A. (1979) 'Implementation as evolution', in J.L. Pressman and A. Wildavsky (eds.) Implementation: How Great Expectations in Washington Are Dashed in Oakland, University of California Press, Berkeley, California

MAPLIN (1981) Managing the Manpower Future, HMSO, London

Marsh, G. and Kaim-Caudle, P. (1976) Team Care in General Practice, Croom Helm, London

Maynard, A. and Walker, A. (1977) 'A critical survey of medical manpower planning in Britain', Social and Economic Administration, Vol. 11, No. 1, pp. 52-75

Mead, J., Crawford, M. and Wells, J. (1985) 'Training for helpers', Occupational Therapy, July, pp. 211-14

Bibliography

Mejia, A. (1978) 'The health manpower process', in T.L. Hall and A. Mejia (eds.) Health Manpower Planning: Principles, Methods and Issues, WHO, Geneva, ch. 1

Melia, K. (1983) 'Doing nursing and being professional', Nursing Times, 1 June, pp. 28-30

Mercer, G. and Long, A.F. (1981) 'The state and managerial innovation. A case study from the British health service', Scandanavian Journal of Social Medicine, Supplementum 28, pp. 263-274

Mercer, J. (1981) 'Health care and remedial professionalism', Health Services Manpower Review, Vol. 7, No. 1, pp. 11-13

Metcalfe, D. (1982) 'Flexible doctoring', The Health Services, 14 May, p. 20

Ministry of Health (1962) A Hospital Plan for England and Wales, Cmnd. 1604, HMSO, London

Ministry of Health (1966) Health and Welfare: The Development of Community Care, HMSO, London

Mittler, P. (1979) People not Patients, Methuen, London

Morrin, H.A. (1982) 'Are we in danger of extinction?', Midwives Chronicle and Nursing Notes, January, p.17

Morris, P. (1969) Put Away, Routledge and Kegan Paul, London

Mourin, K. (1980) 'The role of the practice nurse', Journal of the Royal College of General Practitioners, Vol. 30, February, pp. 75-77

National Audit Office (1985a) National Health Service: Hospital Based Medical Manpower, Report by the Comptroller and Auditor General, HMSO, London

National Audit Office (1985b) National Health Service: Control of Nursing Manpower, Report by the Comptroller and Auditor General, HMSO, London

Newson, K. (1982) 'The future of midwifery', Midwifery, Health Visitor and Community Nurse, Vol. 18, December, pp. 520-30

Noack, H. (ed.) (1980) Medical Education and Primary Health Care, Croom Helm, London

Nuffield Foundation (1980) Dental Education: Report of a Committee of Inquiry, The Nuffield Foundation, London

Ovretveit, J. (1985) 'Medical dominance and the development of autonomy in physiotherapy', Sociology of Health and Illness, Vol. 7, No. 1, pp. 76-93

Parkhouse, J. (1979) Medical Manpower in Britain, Churchill Livingstone, Edinburgh

Bibliography

Parkhouse, J. (1986) 'Manpower: compendium of deliberate mistakes', British Medical Journal, Vol. 292, 10 May, pp. 1286-7

Parkhouse, J., Campbell, M.G. and Parkhouse, H.F. (1983) 'Career preferences of doctors qualifying in 1974-80: a comparison of pre-registration findings', Health Trends, Vol. 15, No. 2, pp.29-35

Parkhouse, J. and O'Brien, N. (1984) 'Medical and dental training and staffing in a region - the long and short of it', British Medical Journal, Vol. 288, 9 June, pp. 1773-1775

Pearse, I. and Crocker, L. (1943) The Peckham Experiment. A Study in the Living Structure of Society, Allen and Unwin, London

Petch, R. (1981) 'The role of the DHSS', in A.F. Long and G. Mercer (eds.) Manpower Planning in the National Health Service, Gower, Farnborough, ch. 6

Plank, M. (1982) Teams for Mentally Handicapped People, Campaign for Mentally Handicapped People, London

Platt Report (1959) The Welfare of Children in Hospital, HMSO, London

Platt Report (1961) Report of the Joint Working Party on the Medical Staffing Structure in the Hospital Services, HMSO, London

Pledger, G. (1984) 'Planning roles', Health and Social Services Journal, 12 July, p. 823

Pollitt, C. (1985) 'Measuring performance: a new system for the National Health Service', Policy and Politics, Vol. 13, No. 1, pp. 1-15

Poulton, K. (1985) 'The dynamics of change', Senior Nurse, Vol. 3, No. 5, pp. 13-16

Pursur, R.G. (1984) 'Future relationships between DHAs and FPCs', Hospital and Health Services Review, July, pp. 167-170

Pursur, R.G. (1986) 'A brave new world for the family practitioner services?' in D.P. Gray (ed.) The Medical Annual 1986, pp. 224-235

Rathwell, T. (1984) 'Health services planning: observations on the relationship between theory and practice', in M. Clarke (ed.) Planning and Analysis in Health Care Systems, Pion, London, pp. 119-141

Rathwell, T. and Barnard, K. (1985) 'Health services performance in Great Britain', in A.F. Long and S. Harrison (eds.) Health Services Performance: Effectiveness and Efficiency, Croom Helm, London, ch. 6

Bibliography

Rathwell, T., Long, A.F. and Harrison, S. (1985) 'Scenarios for health manpower development: a conceptual framework', unpublished paper, Nuffield Centre, University of Leeds

Reedy, B.L. (1977) 'The health team' in J. Fry (ed.) Trends in General Practice, British Medical Journal, London, ch. 6

Reedy, B.L. (1980) 'Teamwork in primary health care: a conspectus', in J. Fry (ed.) Primary Care, Heinemann, London, ch. 6

Reedy, B.L. (1981) 'Discrepancies in the perceptions of a structural relationship for teamwork', Nursing Times, Occasional Papers 77, pp. 89-96

Regional Personnel Officer/Manpower Resourcing Interest Group (1984) Manpower and the Planning Process: A Checklist for District Personnel Officers, DHSS, London

Remedial Therapist (1984) Editorial, 14 December, p. 1

Rogers, R. (1986) 'No room at the top', Senior Nurse, Vol. 4, No. 1, p. 5

Rookes, P. (1982) 'How many health visitors?', Nursing Times, 1 December, pp. 2043-45

Roten, A., Barnoon, S., and Prywes, M. (1985) 'Is integration of health services and manpower development possible? The Beer Sheva case study', Health Policy, 5, pp. 223-239

Rowden, R. (1985) 'A climate of fear', Nursing Mirror, Vol. 151, No. 18, pp. 25-26

Royal College of General Practitioners (1972) The Future General Practitioner: Learner and Teacher, British Medical Journal, London

Royal College of General Practitioners (1981) 'What sort of doctor?', Journal of the Royal College of General Practitioners, Vol. 31, pp. 698-702

Royal College of General Practitioners (1985) What Sort of Doctor? Assessing Quality of Care in General Practice, Report from General Practice 23, RCGP, London

Royal College of Nursing (1984) Training Needs of Practice Nurses, RCN, London

Royal College of Nursing Commission on Nursing Education (1985) The Education of Nurses: A New Dispensation (Judge Report), RCN, London

Royal Commission on the National Health Service (1979) Report, Cmnd. 7615, HMSO, London

Ruston, G. (1985) 'Centres of conflicting interests', Health and Social Services Journal, 7 February, pp. 156-158

Sanders, D.J., Stone, V., Fowler, G. and Maraillier,
J. (1986) 'Practice nurses and antismoking
education',British Medical Journal, Vol. 292, 8
February, pp. 381-382
Sanders, G. and O'Brien, M. (1985) 'A regional
manpower plan for community medicine', Vol. 7,
pp. 116-121
Schofield, T. and Hasler, J. (1984) 'Approval of
trainers and training practices in the Oxford
region', British Medical Journal, Vol. 288, pp.
538-540, 612-614, 688-689
Scottish Home and Health Department (1984) The Role of
the Paramedical Professions, HMSO, London
Scott Samuel, A. (1984) 'Need for primary health care:
an objective indicator', British Medical
Journal, Vol. 28, 11 February, pp. 457-458
Seebohm Report (1968) Committee on Local Authority and
Allied Personal Social Services Report, Cmnd.
3703, HMSO, London
Short Report (1981) Medical Education, Vols. 1-4,
HMSO, London
Spens Report (1948) Report of the Inter-Departmental
Committee on the Remuneration of Consultants and
Specialists, Cmnd. 7420, HMSO, London
Stilwell, B. (1982a) 'The nurse practitioner at work.
1 Primary Care', Nursing Times, Vol. 78,
27 October, pp. 1799-1803
Stilwell, B. (1982b) 'The nurse practitioner at
work. 2 The American Experience', Nursing Times,
Vol. 78, 3 November, pp. 1859-60
Stilwell, B. (1982c) 'The nurse practitioner at
work. 3 Clinical Practice', Nursing Times, Vol.
78, 10 November, pp. 1909-1910
Stilwell, B. (1984) 'The nurse in practice', Nursing
Mirror, Vol. 158, 23 May, pp. 17-19
Stocking, B. (1979) 'Confusion or control? Manpower
in the complementary professions' in G.
McLachlan, B. Stocking and R.F.A. Shegog (eds.)
Patterns for Uncertainty? Planning for the
Greater Medical Profession, Nuffield Provincial
Hospitals Trust, London
Stocking, B. (1980) 'The next decade: a critique of
the CPSM Report', Health Services Manpower
Review, Vol. 6, No. 2, pp. 11-14
Stocking, B. (1985) Initiative and Inertia, Nuffield
Provincial Hospitals Trust, London
Strong, P. (1986) 'A new-modelled medicine? Comments
on the WHO's Regional Strategy for Europe',
Social Science and Medicine, Vol. 22, No. 2, pp.
193-99

Bibliography

Teviot Report (1946) <u>Final Report of the Inter</u>
<u>Department Committee on Dentistry</u>, Cmnd. 6727,
Ministry of Health, HMSO, London
Todd, G. (1983) 'The challenge of medical manpower
planning', <u>Health Services Manpower Review</u>, Vol.
9, No. 2, pp. 3-6
Todd, G. (1985) 'Towards a rational plan for manpower
needs', <u>Health and Social Service Journal</u>, 18
April, pp. 478-479
Todd, G., O'Brien, M. and Gooding, D. (1985) 'Career
structure - the modern doctor dilemma', <u>British</u>
<u>Medical Journal</u>, Vol. 291, 14 September,
pp. 755-756
Todd, J.N. and Coyne, A-M. (1985) 'Medical manpower:
a district model', <u>British Medical Journal</u>, Vol.
291, 5 October, pp. 984-985
Todd Report (1968) <u>Royal Commission on Medical</u>
<u>Education Report</u>, Cmnd 3569, HMSO, London
Towler, J. (1982) 'Midwives units wishful thinking and
reality', <u>Midwives Chronicle and Nursing Notes</u>,
January, pp. 3-5
Towell, D. and Harries, C. (eds.) (1979) <u>Innovation in</u>
<u>Patient Care</u>, Croom Helm, London
Turton, P. (1985) 'Jill of all trades?', <u>Nursing Times</u>,
25 September, pp. 24-25
United Kingdom Central Council - Educational Policy
Advisory Committee (1985a) <u>Introducing Project</u>
<u>2000</u>, Project Paper 1, UKCC, London
United Kingdom Central Council (1985b) <u>The Leaver:</u>
<u>Student Status Revisited</u>, Project Paper 2, UKCC,
London
United Kingdom Central Council (1985c) <u>One-Two-Three:</u>
<u>How Many Levels of Nurse Should There Be?</u>,
Project Paper 3, UKCC, London
United Kingdom Central Council (1985d) <u>The Enrolled</u>
<u>Nurse</u>, Project Paper 4, UKCC, London
United Kingdom Central Council (1985e) <u>Redrawing the</u>
<u>Boundaries?</u>, Project Paper 5, UKCC, London
United Kingdom Central Council (1985f) <u>Facing the</u>
<u>Future</u>, Project Paper 6, UKCC, London
United Kingdom Central Council (1986) <u>Project 2000</u>,
UKCC, London
Vaughan, D.H. (1982) 'Changing gear: problems of
selecting appropriate staffing ratios', <u>British</u>
<u>Medical Journal</u>, Vol. 284, 15 May, pp. 1498-1499
Walker, R.O. <u>et al</u> (1965) 'Dentistry in the United
Kingdom', <u>British Dental Journal</u>, 17 August, pp.
139-146; and 7 September, pp. 184-192
Walton, H.J. (1985) 'Primary health care in European
medical education: a survey', <u>Medical Education</u>,
Vol. 19, pp. 167-188

Bibliography

Watkin, B. (1978) The National Health Service: The First Phase, Allen and Unwin, London

Weisfeld, N. (1984) 'The national commission for health certifying agencies: an introduction', Health Policy, 4, pp. 63-79

Wilcox, R. (1984) 'Improving the FPC's planning and development role', Family Practitioner Services, Vol. 11, No. 5, pp. 101-102

Wilkin, D. (1979) Caring for the Mentally Handicapped Child, Croom Helm, London

Wilkin, D., and Metcalfe, D.H. (1984) 'List size and patient contact in general medical practice', British Medical Journal, Vol. 289, 1 December, pp 1501-1505

Williams, J. (1984) 'Funding for physiotherapy', Health and Social Service Journal, 20 September, pp. 1113

Williams, J. (1985) 'Who should hold the budget?' Health and Social Service Journal, 12 September, pp. 1128-1129

Williams, J., Parry, E. Deeley, W., Atherton, M. and Lauder, N. (1981) 'Paramedical services: low cost efficiency', Health and Social Service Journal, 10 April, pp. 418-419

Willink Report (1957) Report of the Committee to Consider the Future Numbers of Medical Practitioners and the Appropriate Intake of Medical Students, HMSO, London

Willmott, J. (1980) 'Specialists in birth', Nursing Mirror, 8 July, pp. 34-35

Wistow, G. (1985) 'Community care for the mentally handicapped: disappointing progress', in A. Harrison and J. Gretton (eds.) Health Care UK 1985, Chartered Institute of Public Finance and Accountancy, London, pp. 69-78

Wood Report (1947) Report of the Working Party on the Recruitment and Training of Nurses, Ministry of Health, HMSO, London

World Health Organization (1948) Constitution, WHO, Geneva

World Health Organization (1978) Primary Health Care, Report of the International Conference on Primary Health Care, Alma-Ata, USSR, WHO, Geneva

World Health Organization (1979) Formulating Strategies for Health-For-All by the Year 2000, WHO, Geneva

World Health Organization (1981) Managerial Process for National Health Development: Guiding Principles, WHO, Geneva

Bibliography

World Health Organization (1985a) Primary Health Care in Industrialised Countries, EURO Reports and Studies No. 95, WHO, Copenhagen

World Health Organization (1985b) Targets for Health for All, WHO, Copenhagen

World Health Organization (1985c) Medical Specialisation in Relation to Health Needs, WHO, Copenhagen

World Health Organization (1986) Implementation of Health Manpower Policies, Plans and Programmes: Future Perspectives, Report of an Inter-Regional Consultation, Jakarta, Indonesia, 15-19 October, 1984, WHO/EDUC/86.186, WHO, Geneva

Yates, J. and Davidge, M. (1984) 'Can you measure performance?', British Medical Journal, Vol. 288, No. 1, pp. 1935-1936

Index